Health Care Computing

Health Care Computing

A survival guide for PC users

PHILIP BURNARD

School of Nursing Studies
University of Wales College of Medicine
Heath Park
Cardiff
UK

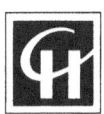

SPRINGER-SCIENCE+BUSINESS MEDIA, B.V.

Distributed in the USA and Canada by Singular Publishing Group Inc.,
4284 41st Street, San Diego, California 92105

First edition 1995

Originally published by Chapman & Hall in 1995

Typeset in 10.5/13 pt Palatino by Best-set Typesetter Ltd., Hong Kong

ISBN 978-0-412-60530-7   ISBN 978-1-4899-3234-1 (eBook)
DOI 10.1007/978-1-4899-3234-1

A catalogue record for this book is available from the British Library

∞ Printed on permanent acid-free text paper, manufactured in
accordance with ANSI/NISO Z39.48-1992 and ANSI/NISO Z39.48-1984
(Permanence of Paper).

For Sally, Aaron and Rebecca

Contents

Acknowledgements

All trade marks of software, companies and publishers are acknowledged. Thanks, as ever, to my son, Aaron, who has taught me a considerable amount about computers and has helped me to survive with a personal computer. Thanks also to Marianne Talberg of the University of Tampere for allowing me to use her personal library of books and papers on computing in Helsinki, Finland.

Particular thanks go to Computer Manuals, 50 James Road, Tyseley, Birmingham B11 2BA for supplying review copies of many of the books that are referred to in this book. Acknowledgements go to the Editor of *Windows User* for permission to reproduce, in Chapters 2 and 5, details from Mark Stephens' article 'The Happy Shopper', from the December 1993 edition of that magazine.

Introduction

Most health professionals have to use computers – at least some of the time. Frequently, those computers are **personal** computers – the generic name for the ones that are variously known as 'IBM compatible' or 'IBM clones' or just PCs. This separates them out from certain other makes such as the Apple Macintosh, the Amstrad dedicated word-processor, the Atari, Amiga and a number of others. This book is about PCs.

When you need information about your computer when you are busy, you don't want to have to wade through piles of manuals to find what you need. You often need a fairly straightforward piece of information – now. Computers can be infuriating. When they are up and running properly, they can save time and help you to be more productive. When something goes wrong, they can be extremely frustrating. Once you have called in someone else to fix your problem, it is often apparent that the answer to your problem was only a few keystrokes away. This book aims at supplying you with small chunks of information that can aid your productivity, get you out of awkward corners and help you to become more at home with your PC. It has been my experience – as a health care lecturer and as a regular computer user – that you need to develop a certain baseline of confidence in working with them. At first, you are almost afraid to touch the keyboard unless anything goes wrong. Then, you become more skilled in using the machine but still need to call on someone else to help you out. Finally, you build up a stock of knowledge that allows you to work out most things for yourself. In the end, there is, of course, a limited number of things that can go wrong with a PC. This book offers you information – some basic and some not so basic – that can help you to understand aspects of your computer and figure out how to manage on your own.

With the idea of giving you maximum information in a fairly small amount of space and to make that information more digestible, the book is made up of a series of chapters containing tips, traps and help boxes.

Tip

Each tip section contains a discrete piece of information about the topic in question. All of these tips are indexed at the back of the book.

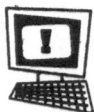

Trap

Each trap section highlights a potential problem and suggests ways of overcoming it. Like the tips, these are indexed at the back of the book.

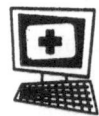

Help

'Help' sections offer more details about specific issues. They offer background detail and further information about the topic contained in the chapter. Refer to them when you need to go deeper into a topic.

Computers can be fun as well as infuriating. Many of the tips in this book are of the sort that will help you to speed up your work and make your PC run more efficiently. These days, personal computers are extremely powerful and it is important to use that power as effectively as possible. It is not uncommon to find people using only a small percentage of the capacity of their computers simply because they are not set up properly. It is also possible to come across people who use them as glorified typewriters and who work in ways that are more suited to a typewriter. Again, there are tips about getting the most out of your machine when preparing documents, reports, articles and books. It is said that PCs are used far more for wordprocessing than for any other function. It pays to use that wordprocessing power effectively.

Each chapter of the book ends with a detailed review of one or two other books related to the chapter topic. At the end of the book, I have included a list of some other books about computing.

This book can be read on its own or as a companion volume to my previous title *Personal Computing for Health Professionals*, also published by Chapman & Hall, which offers a broad introduction to personal computing. In this one, I have purposely adopted the concise approach to identifying information about computing. The book is aimed at the newcomer and also at the person who has had some experience of computing but who wants to know more.

The computing world is changing rapidly. Processors, printers and programs alter almost daily. Indeed, some software companies have stopped quoting a 'recommended price' for their products, knowing that such figures would quickly be grossly undercut in the market place. Given the rapid changes in pricing policy, I have not quoted any prices. I have also aimed at discussing only those programs that are fairly widely available and seem likely to remain current for a few years – even if they are updated at regular intervals. Programs like *WordPerfect* and *Word for Windows*, for example, have been in production for a number of years and it seems unlikely that they will suddenly disappear.

Computers can free health professionals to do what they were trained and educated to do. Health care educators can use them to enhance their teaching methods and to help their students to learn more effectively. Managers and those in the clinical field can also benefit from their capacity to store and recall information rapidly. We cannot avoid computers and we may as well make the most of them. I hope that this book aids that process and makes personal computing easier and, perhaps, more interesting.

WHO IS THIS BOOK FOR?

This is for anyone who is using a personal computer (IBM compatible or 'clone'). It assumes that any health professional using it will have got to the stage of starting the computer and beginning to use it. Thus it is for 'beginners and intermediate' users. These include the following groups:

- Students in the health care professions;
- Managers;

- Educators, trainers and staff in college and university departments;
- Those working in private health care institutions;
- Clinical and field workers;
- Those in the quality assurance and audit fields;
- Researchers;
- Network managers;
- Home computer users.

WHAT IS IN THE BOOK?

As we have noted above, this book is made up of readily assimilated information about a variety of topics related to using PCs.

Chapter 1 is all about buying a personal computer. It covers where to buy and what sort of machine to consider. Chapter 2 covers buying software and points to some of the problems of selecting and using programs. Chapter 3 is about setting up your computer and making it run optimally. Chapter 4 considers one of the most important parts of the PC world: the disk operating system (DOS). Chapter 5 is about *Windows* – one of the most widely used platforms on which software is run. Chapter 6 discusses issues related to organizing and classifying your computer files. Chapter 7 considers a range of shortcuts and hints about using a wordprocessor on the PC.

Chapter 8 identifies problems and suggestions concerning the use of databases both in the health care professions and in the home. Chapter 9 identifies some of the best ways of working with writing projects and how best to design documents. Chapter 10 offers practical suggestions for organizing research using a PC.

The book closes with an appendix which summarizes important details of the Data Protection Act 1984 – an Act that all computer users should have some knowledge of.

Tips and traps in buying a personal computer

Health care professionals not only need to use computers: at some point many of them have to buy one. This chapter offers tips and traps related to the business of buying a computer. The buying may be for personal use or for use in an office, clinic or community setting. If you have never bought a computer before, you are advised to seek help from a computer expert at the point of sale. Take one with you if you are buying a computer. Most health authorities, colleges and universities have a computing department and they will usually advise on the sort of machine to buy.

Tip

Do you want to use *Windows*? If so, you need the right sort of computer.

Windows is a software application made by Microsoft. First, you have the computer. Then you have the **disk operating system** (DOS), sitting between the programs you use and the computer. Third, you can add *Windows*, 'on top' of DOS and this allows you to take advantage of the power offered by modern computers to do various things, including the following:

- Use a **graphical interface**. This means that, instead of being presented with an almost blank screen when you turn on the computer, you are offered a series of small pictures (**icons**) which represent your programs. When you double-click the left hand mouse button when the mouse pointer is on one of these icons, the program starts. All *Windows* programs make considerable use of the mouse and encourage you to 'point and shoot' rather than to remember complicated keystroke routines.

- Run a number of programs at the same time. This is known as **multitasking**. Working in this way, you can quickly switch between your wordprocessor and your database. You can also cut and paste information straight out of one program into another.

- Learn the standard *Windows* format. Most *Windows* programs use the same screen layout and a similar set of drop-down menus at the top of the screen. This means that once you have learned one *Windows* program, it is usually easy to learn another.

- Make full use of the memory capabilities and the power of up-to-date personal computers.

You will find more about *Windows* in Chapter 5. Suffice it to say at this point that if you want to use *Windows* (and most people seem to) you need to buy a computer powerful enough to run it. *Windows* takes up a lot of the power of the main computer chip, a lot of memory and *Windows* programs tend to occupy a lot of space on the hard disk. Here are two sample specifications of PCs for running *Windows*:

Base machine

Processor:	486SX 25MHx
Memory:	4Mb
Video (monitor):	Super VGA
Floppy disk:	One 3½"
Hard disk:	80–100Mb

Power machine

Processor:	486DX 50Mhz or Pentium
Memory:	8–16Mb
Video (monitor):	Accelerated Super VGA
Floppy disk:	One 3½"
Hard disk:	200–300Mb

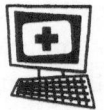

Help

Do you need a Pentium chip?

The newest and fastest processor available at the time of writing is the '506' or Pentium chip. The temptation, if you or your budget can run to it, is always to consider the newest and fastest processing chip.

However, the Pentium chip is not a necessity for every health care user. Kennedy (1993) identifies five reasons why you might need a Pentium chip:

1. You run CPU-intensive applications, such as programming, graphic design or desktop publishing.
2. You use applications that rely on complex floating-point calculations, such as spreadsheets.
3. You're developing sophisticated multimedia applications that incorporate full-motion video, sound and video capture.
4. You run a variety of x86 software and want backward compatibility but with better-than-486 performance.
5. You're ready to switch to 32-bit NT applications (NT is a type of **network operating system**).

If you do not fall into one of these categories, Kennedy concludes that you are likely to be better off with a 486 or lesser processor.

Tip

You don't necessarily need a state-of-the-art computer.

The most expensive computers are always going to be the latest and fastest. An 'old fashioned' computer is often one that was state-of-the-art only two years previously. If your computing needs are fairly straightforward and involve mostly wordprocessing, you can save a lot of money by buying a computer that contains an 'older' processing chip. If, for example, you plan to use mostly DOS programs, a 286 processor in a computer containing a 40Mb hard disk will often be quite adequate. It will also be available for a very reasonable sum of money. If you buy this sort of machine, however, check that you can upgrade it if you later find that you need to. Faster machines are nearly always necessary if you plan to do a lot of graphical work or to run a large and complicated statistics or database program. On the other hand, I currently have a research assistant who runs *Word for Windows* on a 286 computer and has no problems at all with it – although the computer does have 4Mb of RAM.

Draw up a checklist of the specification of the computer that you need.

Items to note and check are the follwoing.

- Make and model of the computer you want;
- Main chip specification (386SX, 486SX, etc.);
- Speed of the processor, in megahertz (MHz);
- Size and number of floppy drives;
- Hard disk size;
- Amount of RAM (random access memory) required (for *Windows* you will need at least 2Mb. 4Mb is better and 8–16Mb is recommended);
- Operating system and *Windows* included?
- Other software bundled with the computer;
- Is a mouse included in the price?
- Type of casing: desktop or tower;
- Details of guarantee and warranty;
- Price, including VAT and postage;
- Cost of any other extras.

Tip

If you work in a college or university department or if you are a student, you may be able to obtain a special 'educational' price when buying a computer.

Many companies that sell computers operate a two-tier system of pricing. There is one price for the general public and for business and another for the educational sector. You may have to show evidence of being a student or order your computer on college-headed paper to take advantage of this price. If you can obtain an educational discount, it is always worthwhile. Indeed, you may want to deal only with those companies that do offer this service. The amount of discount can be considerable and varies from company to company. If you are buying for a government or educational institution, the order may also be VAT exempt. Again, check on the policy of both the institution for whom you work and the company with which you are placing your order. These VAT exemptions are not usually available to private individuals. Again, there are usually special ways of ordering equipment that is VAT exempt.

Tip

Read the computer magazines to get a clear idea about pricing.

The computer market is one of the most volatile. Prices of chips are usually dropping all the time. This affects the price of the computer you buy. One of the best ways of keeping abreast of changes in the prices of computers (and software) is to read one or more of the computer magazines. The following is a shortlist of such publications in the UK:

Computer Shopper
PC Answers
PC Today
Personal Computer World
Windows User
PC Direct
PC Format

These magazines are also a good way of getting acquainted with a range of software; many include a 'free' disk on the front cover. Some of them contain **shareware** (discussed in the next chapter), while others contain sample programs that will run for a few weeks to enable you to evaluate them. Others, however, are much more generous and contain complete, commercial programs. These are usually ones that were published a couple of years previously and have been overtaken by new models. They are, however, complete and uncut and excellent value.

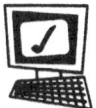

Tip

Buying through the post can be a cost effective way of buying a computer.

Buying through the post means that overheads and middlemen are cut out. This usually results in far lower prices being offered by mail order companies than by High Street shops. Again, access to these companies is often through the computer magazines. Most companies will accept telephone orders, with a credit card and most will accept faxed orders on company or institute order forms. Big companies, like Dell and Elonex, have gained a reputation for their excellent service in the mail order field. You need to be careful, though; a number of mail order companies have gone bankrupt in the last few years. Check with someone in the know before buying by this route but do consider this approach – it is nearly always the cheapest option.

Tip

Consider, too, the PC supermarkets.

A variety of PC supermarkets has sprung up in the UK, following the trend in the States. These allow you to see what you are buying and yet are able to offer a considerable discount when compared with the High Street shops. They are not usually as cheap as mail order companies but you have the advantage of seeing before you buy and of having somewhere local to return faulty goods to.

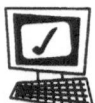

Tip

Make sure that you have the appropriate warranty for your needs.

There are usually two forms of warranty offered when computers are sold: 'back to base' and 'on site'. With a back to base warranty, you are responsible for packaging up the computer and returning it to the company if the machine goes wrong. With an on site warranty, the company has an arrangement with a servicing organization who will come and repair the computer in your office or your home. On site agreements are usually more expensive but are often worth the peace of mind.

Tip

Be clear about what you are buying: think before you buy.

There are various pitfalls to be overcome when buying a computer and it is usually best to have somebody to help you in the decision making and buying process. Most health authorities, colleges and university departments have one or more computer experts on hand to help you in this way. It is worth considering the following points that Magee (1993) offers:

1. Check the specifications of the machine and the software you want against your needs. If you are buying for business purposes, take advice from colleagues in the same field.
2. Compare prices for similar specified machines in the High Street, through superstores and buying directly through magazines like *Computer Buyer*.
3. Check the details of the after-sales support. How comprehensive is the agreement? Will the company come out and fix your machine the same day? This is important if your business relies on the computer you've bought.
4. If you're buying by mail order, satisfy yourself that the company is financially stable by calling them and asking them for references from satisfied customers, how long they've been in business and so on. If you're in any doubt, put them to one side.
5. When you've found the PC and/or software you think are suitable, buy a number of magazines that carry reviews and compare what they say about the products.

Tip

If your computing needs are modest, you may not need a PC at all.

If all you need is something on which to produce basic, textual documents – letters and perhaps an essay or two – the Amstrad Notepad may be sufficient for your needs.

The Amstrad Notepad offers remarkable value for money. It is a simple, notebook computer that runs on four AA batteries. It contains a good wordprocessor (a version of *Protext*), a diary, a calculator and a set of alarms. It is the ideal portable computer for the person on the move and it costs less than £200. More than that, the batteries have a life of about 30 hours and this beats all of competition. On the down side, the screen is fairly small and not backlit so people who are used to more sophisticated machines will take a little time to get used to this. On the other hand, the whole machine weighs only a couple of pounds and easily fits into a briefcase. The computer has no hard disk and files are stored within the computer when it is switched off. Standard memory is only 64K but further storage is obtainable as RAM cards. I have found the Notepad an ideal computer for writing when travelling. It is extremely easy to use, has a good keyboard and files from it can be transferred to a full PC.

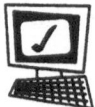

Tip

Remember to budget for a printer when you plan your computer buying.

With certain integrated wordprocessing machines like the Amstrad, the computer, printer and wordprocessing software come together as a complete bundle. This is not the case with PCs. First, you buy the computer, then the printer and then the software. All three elements have to be costed separately. It used to be said that you should decide on the software you need first and then decide on a suitable computer and printer. Today, much of the *Windows* software uses similar sorts of computing power and this is no longer the imperative that it was. You must, however, decide on what sort of printer you need.

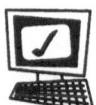

Tip

Know the difference between the different types of printer.

There are three main types of printer: the dot matrix, the inkjet and the laser. All three work in different sorts of ways, cost different amounts of money and can be used for different purposes. However, all of them will reproduce text and can be used for printing out wordprocessed documents. What distinguishes them is both price and print quality; the two tend to go together. Whatever the type of printer, the more you pay for it, the better the print quality. Placed on a spectrum, the dot matrix printers tend to be the cheapest and offer the poorest quality of printout while the laser printers tend to be the most expensive and offer the highest quality printout.

Dot matrix printers work via a series of pins pushing against a 'typewriter' ribbon. The 'matrix' is the set of pins used in the process. Dot matrix printers tend to be slow and noisy but also tend to be very reliable. They are less complicated to run than the other two sorts and less expensive to service.

Inkjet printers work by forcing a fine spray of ink onto the page in the shape of letters, characters or graphics. They tend to be very quiet in operation and their price is beginning to drop to equal those of the dot matrix printers. They can produce print quality almost equalling some laser printers but they tend to need ink refills fairly regularly and these can be comparatively expensive. Various companies supply kits for refilling the inkjet cartridges. Inkjets are probably the best low cost option for the home user or the small health care department. It is also possible to buy inkjet printers that offer colour output.

Laser printers offer the highest quality printout. This can rival book and journal quality printing and laser output is used by some publishers for 'camera-ready copy' – text that is supplied by the author, ready to be photographed for final printing. Laser printers are fast, fairly quiet and the smaller ones are competitively priced. Toner cartridges for different machines vary widely in price. When you are exploring the options in the laser printer market, consider the cost of these cartridges. Replacements can sometimes be more than £100. The cartridges also vary in the number of sheets that they will print. Again, check expected output per cartridge before you buy.

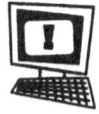

Trap

Don't automatically assume that you need a laser printer.

Although laser printers produce the highest quality printout, the inkjet and even the dot matrix can be more than adequate for many computer users. If, for example, you are a social worker who needs to produce two or three written reports and some letters every week, your needs might best be served by an inkjet printer. If you need to print out continuous stationery (printed forms that are joined together and separated by tearing apart), the dot matrix printer is likely to be your only option. Also, for heavy duty work, a dot matrix printer can turn out to be the most reliable option. Most laser printers cannot handle very long print runs and demand a 'rest period' every so often. Indeed, some have a built-in facility to switch themselves off if the expected output for a given period is exceeded. Laser printers cannot be run continuously, over a series of 24 hour periods. Dot matrix printers usually can and are often used to service large networks of computers in health care colleges and university departments. Also, dot matrix printers are ideal for printing out labels – a function that is quite difficult to perform with a laser or inkjet printer.

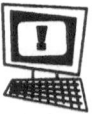

Trap

Dot matrix printers usually do not allow you to print a wide range of fonts or typefaces.

If you need to use a Roman typeface (this book is printed in such a face), you usually cannot use a dot matrix printer. Most printers of this sort limit you to various versions of the Courier typeface, which looks very like the output from a typewriter. On the other hand, this is often quite adequate for correspondence. In fact some people prefer the look of the Courier font for reports and correspondence.
Examples:

```
This is an example of a Courier font. It looks very
like the typeface used in most typewriters.
```

This is an example of a Times Roman font. It is one of the most frequently used of the fonts supplied with *Windows* and it – or a variant of it – is frequently used in the printing trade.

Tip

Think big.

In the first tip in this chapter, two specifications were identified. It is important to check whether or not either of these conform to any sort of state-of-the-art specification. Indeed, making such a comparison with the sorts of computers that are being used when you read this book will serve as an index of the degree and speed of change in the computer world. Computing is still developing at a rapid rate. What was considered a powerful machine two years ago is now thought of as almost unusable by many people. Think big. Buy the most highly specified machine that you can, if you have any plans to expand in the future. If you are certain that you will never need to do anything more than wordprocessing with your computer then this is not so important. However, computers can change the way you work and as you find more use for them, you will find yourself using different sorts of programs. This, in turn, will mean that you use more and more hard disk space. As a rule, buy the largest hard disk and the largest amount of memory (RAM) that you can afford.

Tip

Consider what sort of peripheral devices you might need.

First, it is essential to make provision for **backing up** your hard disk. This means, as we shall see in a later chapter, that you should have a copy of everything that is on your hard disk, on a different medium. In the past, this used to mean on floppy disks. However, the situation has changed: hard disks are frequently 100Mb or more in size and as such, cannot readily be backed up to floppies. One of the most economical and rapid media for containing a copy of your hard disk is the **tape streamer**. This is a small device like a tape recorder that plugs into your computer or is contained within the main box. The tape streamer is accompanied by backup software and it allows you to backup:

1. the total contents of your hard disk;
2. some of the files;
3. just those files that have changed since the last backup.

If you are buying a new computer, you may want to consider buying one with an integrated tape streamer.

As software packages grow in size, so software companies are beginning to supply programs on compact disks. These are virtually the same disks as the ones used in the music industry but they contain computer data instead of music. The point about compact disks, in the computer world, is that they can be read by the computer but not written to. In other words, you can open and copy files from the disk but you cannot write new information to it. For this reason, they are known as **CD-ROMs** (Compact Disk: Read Only Memory). To use them, you need a CD-ROM player. Like tape streamers, CD-ROM players come either as integral units or as add-on devices. Again, you may want to consider one of these when buying a new machine. If you use your computer for desktop publishing or for graphics work, you can buy CD-ROMs full of typefaces and graphics in the form of **clip art**. Clip art is small pictures and pieces of graphics that can be incorporated into your own work. There is also a range of dictionaries and books available in CD-ROM format.

Finally, you may want to consider a **scanner**. A scanner is a device that will 'read' graphics and text into your computer, from the printed page. Generally, these machines make a better job of reading graphics and pictures than they do of reading text. Also, separate software is needed for reading text. Scanners and the processes that they use take up very large amounts of hard disk space so, if you are thinking of buying one, you must buy a very large hard disk and also a fast processing chip if you want your scanning to do more than crawl along. Scanning is taking a while to mature but it has considerable implications for the health care professions. It is possible to imagine the day when patient and client forms, notes and reports are routinely scanned into computers. This, in turn, should free the health professional to spend more time in therapeutic work and less in clerical work.

Tip

Do you need multimedia?

The multimedia approach to computing involves working with text, graphics and sound. CD-ROMs are available which make use of these three. There are various CD encyclopaedias which not only allow you to view certain entries but offer you musical or vocal accompaniments as well. Although, at the moment, this is largely a area dominated by games and leisure programs, more serious applications are being developed. *Windows User* magazine (1993) offers the following tips about buying a multimedia computer setup:

1. Always choose a [sound] card capable of playing both wave form sounds and synthesized tunes.
2. Don't forget that you'll also need speakers. For the best in sound quality, an external amplifier is also desirable – check your local hi-fi shop for a bargain.
3. Install all the **Windows** drivers which come with your card – some may have as many as three separate drivers for wave output and internal or external MIDI (musical instrument digital interface).
4. Install both the **Windows** sound drivers and the MCI sound driver – sound programs may require one or both of them.
5. Use the **Windows** speaker driver if you can't afford a sound card, but don't be too surprised if the quality if poor.

Finally, there are two industry standards for the specification of multimedia computer setups, called MPC Level 1 and MPC Level 2. The specifications for the two levels are as follows:

MPC Level I

PC: 386SX, 4Mb memory, 30Mb hard drive
Video: VGA
Windows: 3.0 with multimedia extensions of 3.1
CD-ROM: Single speed drive, capable of transferring 150K per second
Sound: 8 bit sound card, supporting sampling up to 11KHz and MIDI

MPC Level 2

PC: 486SX/25Mhz, 4Mb memory, 160Mb hard disk
Video: VGA display with 65 536 colours
Windows: 3.1
CD-ROM: Double speed drive, capable of transferring 300K per second, XA compatible
Sound: 16 bit sound card, supporting stereo sampling up to 44KHz, microphone, MIDI and joystick ports

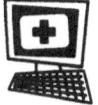

What can you use a multimedia PC for?

Help

Stobie (1994) offers the following list of things you can do with a multimedia PC:

1. Listen to music CDs.
2. Access encyclopaedias and reference material.
3. Load software and clip art more conveniently.
4. View your own photo CD pictures.
5. Capture TV and video images (requires extra hardware).
6. Get enhanced game sound effects.
7. Add voice notes to applications.
8. Control MIDI music devices.
9. Edit audio and video tapes (requires extra hardware).
10. Create multimedia presentations.

Make sure that your computer is upgradable.

If you can't afford lots of RAM and a large hard disk (and even if you can!), make sure that your computer is **upgradable**. Most computers have empty 'slots' into which can be placed other device drivers, motherboards and memory. You must also check that there is room to insert more RAM directly into slots set aside for that purpose.

Finally, you need to know that you can either replace your hard disk with a larger one when you need to or that you can insert a **hard card**. A hard card is a hard disk on a board that is put into one of the spare slots in your computer. This route offers one of the easiest ways of upgrading the hard disk capacity of your computer. Monitors and keyboards are nearly always upgradable.

Consider whether you need a desktop or a notebook computer.

Computers used in offices, clinics and departments are usually 'desktop' computers. That is to say, they consist of a large (or fairly large) box containing the motherboard, the memory chips, the hard disk and the floppy disk driver, the keyboard as a separate unit and the monitor as a separate item that usually sits on top of the box. It is important to note that this does not have to be the way a computer system is set up. There is nothing to stop you positioning the box under the desk and using longer leads to the keyboard, monitor and printer. This arrangement can be a tidier one than when everything is on top of the desk.

The alternative to the desktop computer is the **notebook**. This is a small (about the size of an A4 jumbo pad of paper), light computer which contains all of the above elements in one unit. When they first came out, notebook computers could not contain very large hard disks nor very much memory. Also, they always had black and white screens. All this is no longer the case. Notebook computers can match many of the desktop ones in terms of power, speed, memory and data storage capacity. They are also available with colour screens. However, we have yet to see notebook computer screens which match the best of the desktop monitors.

A decision you may have to make is whether to buy a desktop or a notebook or both. It is still true that the keyboards and monitors of desktop machines are generally better in quality and appearance and, in most offices, these are the ones that are more familiar. Many health care professionals find that they value the use of a notebook computer for community visits, for home use and while travelling. Be advised that many airlines are revising their regulations regarding the use of notebook computers inflight. It is not uncommon for their use to be banned within the first and last hours of a flight.

In terms of price, desktop computers still offer the best value. You can buy more computer for the pound if you buy a desktop than is the case with a notebook. On the other hand, a notebook computer does not make your clinic, department or home look so 'technological'. It may be that in many health care areas, the notebook eventually takes over from the desktop.

In a discussion about buying a notebook computer, Moss (1993) offers, amongst others, the following pointers to the purchaser:

- Think about what you'll be using the machine for, then work out exactly the specification you need. On most machines it's difficult or even impossible to fit a larger hard disk.

- Don't be tempted by portables with processors more powerful than you really need. A more powerful CPU (**Central processing unit** – the computer's main chip) won't just cost you money, you'll also pay in terms of reduced battery life.

- Colour screens may seem attractive but do you really need one? Passive matrix colour displays aren't that good and can be hard to read in less than ideal light. Active matrix displays are good, but very expensive. Both will severely add to the drain on your batteries.

- If choosing a mono screen, check how many grey scales are supported. Some older display panels support only 16 and with these, some combinations of foreground and background colours can be unreadable.

- Check what expansion options are available. Applications get larger all the time, so you may want some extra RAM in a year or two's time. And accessories like an external battery pack . . . could prove useful, even if you don't need it now.

- Consider how you'll transfer data between your portable and desktop machines. You may be happy to use floppies, but if you're looking at sub-notebook or palmtop systems (smaller notebooks) then you'll probably need an external drive. The cost of this may not be included in the basic price of the machine.

- Consider buying a machine with a removable hard disk. Not only will this make it easier to lock your data away, but it will allow you to keep hold of it if you ever need to send the machine for repair.

- Is a carrying case included? Not all portables include a case as standard and some of those that are provided don't have a carrying strap.

- Check the warranty arrangements. On site maintenance usually isn't worth having, because it's difficult to repair portables on site and the engineer will probably take the machine away anyway. Worth looking for are guaranteed repair or replacement times with a return to base warranty or an arrangement that provides you with a loan machine while the original is being fixed.

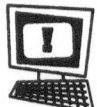

Trap

Try out your keyboard before you buy it.

The keyboard is the most 'subjective' part of the computing system. Some keyboards are like those that used to be found on typewriters and which need considerable strength to press. Others have a 'rubbery' feel to them while still others 'click' fairly loudly and are very precise in action. Which you prefer is very much a question of personal taste. One of the only drawbacks in buying a computer through the post is that you may not be able to try out the keyboard before you buy it. I have found this to be essential. I touch type and have found that I cannot get along with 'rubbery' keyboards: the keys seem to stick and they (or I) produce more errors than when I am using a 'clicky' keyboard. If at all possible, try out a range of keyboards before you buy. If necessary, you can always buy a replacement keyboard for the computer that you buy: keyboards are one of the cheapest components of the computer setup. If you do buy another keyboard, make sure that it is one made for the UK market. It is possible to buy USA keyboards very cheaply but these have a different key layout to the UK ones and may not respond appropriately to the software you are using with the computer.

Gateway produce a keyboard called Anykey which contains another set of function keys to the left of the keyboard and various other extra keys. These keys can be 'programmed' and customized to perform various functions that you use regularly. If you are working with DOS programs in particular, this sort of keyboard can be very useful and can save you time.

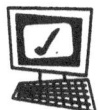

Do you really need a colour monitor?

If your computing needs are modest, if you use your computer mostly for wordprocessing and if you want to assemble the cheapest personal computer package possible, it is a reasonable plan to buy a **mono** monitor. Some computer experts argue that a black and white screen is best for wordprocessing and, in the end, most *Windows* wordprocessors run black type on a white background. I have known at least two health care colleagues who have run their colour monitors in black and white when wordprocessing – clearly a waste of resources in the long run.

On the other hand, don't be spartan for the sake of it. For many programs, a colour monitor brings the program to life and even if little more can be achieved with a colour monitor than with a black and white one, the colour monitor, like the colour television, is preferred by most people.

If you do buy a mono screen, make sure that it is a black and white one. There are still some dark green and bright orange screens available which might suit some users but not others. Check this point particularly if you are buying through the post and responding to an advertisement for a very low cost computing system with a 'mono' screen.

Consider buying a larger monitor if you do a lot of graphics work or desktop publishing.

The standard 14″ screen is adequate for most computing situations. If, however, you do a lot of close, graphical work and need to modify small sections of a drawing or if you want to see the whole of a page of a report on the screen at any given time as you work, you may want to consider buying a larger screen. They are available at 17″, 21″ and 23″. Larger screens also allow you to run your programs at a higher screen resolution. This means that you see more 'dots' to the square inch and thus a clearer, steadier picture. Be careful, though; you need to check that your programs can run with a larger screen and you may need special drivers to enable the computer to work with a non-standard screen. Also, larger screens tend to be expensive.

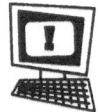

Trap

Check whether or not you need the software that is 'bundled' with your computer.

Many direct mail order suppliers offer 'bundled' software with their products. These can be almost lavish. Some companies, for example, offer state-of-the-art and comprehensive software packages containing wordprocessor, database, spreadsheet and graphics program. Sometimes, combined with the computer, these represent excellent value for money. Other companies, however, bundle rather dated software with their machines – software that may look attractive but which in practice you are unlikely to use. On the principle that you don't get anything for nothing, it is probably best to buy computers on their own and to look around for software bargains in the computer journals. If you do buy bundled software, make sure of your warranty rights and the 'help' service that is not being offered with the software. Also, find out whether or not the software will be preinstalled for you on the hard disk of the computer.

Trap

Check that DOS and *Windows* are included in the total price.

The disk operating system (DOS) is essential for running your computer. Increasingly, as we have seen, *Windows* is becoming a program of choice. Make sure that, at least, DOS is included in the price of your computer. Check, too, that it is installed on your hard disk and that the machine is ready to turn on and use. Find out, as well, whether or not the company supplies *Windows* as a standard installation. Increasingly, machines are being supplied with both of these programs ready installed and 'optimized' for best performance.

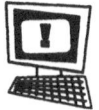

Trap

Check whether or not DOS and *Windows* are preinstalled.

Sometimes, both DOS and *Windows* are supplied on floppy disks but not installed when you buy the computer. If this is the case, you will have to know how to install them. While this is a straightforward enough process, it all adds to the anxiety of someone who is new to computers and who has to rely on the accompanying manuals for guidance. Setting up DOS and *Windows* is discussed in later chapters of this book. If you have to install either of these for the first time, it is wise to have someone who is familiar with computers with you to help.

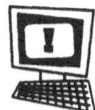

Trap

Bear in mind that most computer magazines quote a price before VAT and postage have been added.

These two 'add-ons' can be considerable. Imagine, for example, a computer and printer package that costs £1500. VAT will be charged at the current rate (which at the time of writing is 17.5%). On top of that, many companies charge quite a considerable amount for delivery. Check both of these figures before you commit yourself to an order.

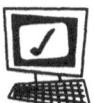

Tip

Could you build your own machine?

One option – and a means of learning all about the insides of computers – is to build your own machine. All the parts are available from companies who regularly advertise in the computer press. In the end, computers are not so complicated: it is the technology involved in the parts that is complicated. One company, Computerlink Training, Wickham House, 10 Cleveland Way, London E1 4TR, offers training courses in building personal computers. During their courses you not only learn how to build one, you actually go ahead and do so.

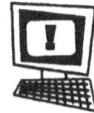

Trap

Building your own computer is not necessarily the cheapest option.

Although the idea of building your own computer may or may not be an attractive option, it is not necessarily the cheapest. When you have bought all the components separately – even from discount dealers – the total cost usually exceeds the price of the most economical, ready-built machines on the market.

Consider leasing as a possible option if you are self-employed.

Tip

If you are self-employed or part of a private or public health care organization, you may want to consider leasing your computing equipment. There are various pros and cons to this procedure but the advantages are these:

1. You can usually offset the whole of the leasing payments against tax.
2. At the end of the leasing period you can often buy the equipment for a nominal sum.
3. You can usually upgrade your equipment on a regular basis without extending the length of your lease.

RECOMMENDED READING

Schueller, U. and Veddeler, H-G. (1992) *Upgrading and Maintaining Your PC*, Abacus. Available from Computer Manuals, 50 James Road, Tyseley, Birmingham B11 2BA. Telephone: 021-706-1188

This book contains essential material for the busy computer user who is trying to keep up with the field. Unfortunately, it is spoilt by some of the heaviest prose I have come across in a computer book. You don't expect computer books to win the Booker Prize but, these days, many of them are very readable. This one is leaden. It is also full of annoying, one-sentence paragraphs that should have been checked by a subeditor. Sometimes, the prose slips into note form.

   For all that, there is some very important and useful information contained in the book. It begins by talking you through the functions of a PC system and describes each element, from the CPU to the hard disk, in some detail. It then illustrates how to use an operating system and how to set up your computer for maximum efficiency. It goes on to show you how to fit new parts. This section is illustrated and offers a step-by-step approach. Here, the pedantic style pays off. You could prop this book open and follow the steps until you had successfully installed a CD-ROM unit. Final chapters offer detailed and important information about troubleshooting and exploring your system. If you can stand the style, there is much of value in this book and anyone who is thinking of 'servicing' his or her own PC would do well to consider buying it.

The book comes with a 'free' disk full of small programs that help you to explore and maximize your system. They include the *System Sleuth Analyzer* which is a toolbox of diagnostic aids rolled into one, easy-to-use software program.

This is a large book of over 600 pages. However, there is a huge amount of padding – almost 200 pages. For whatever reason, the authors have printed out the whole code listing of one of the programs contained on the free disk; 60 pages of code. Another dozen pages offer you a step-by-step account of the program – when all of this is self-explanatory when you run the program itself. Another 100 pages offer you listings of things like 'hard disk parameters', which may be useful to a limited number of people on a very infrequent basis but will not be of much value to the general reader. I would have thought that a better plan would have been to chop the last 200 pages, ditch the 'free' disk and cut £10 off the price of the book.

Upgrading and Maintaining Your PC is not for bedtime reading. It contains specific and seemingly accurate information about various aspects of the PC and it will be an important guide to anyone who wants to take a 'do-it-yourself' approach to computer maintenance. In the end, of course, you won't be buying it for its prose but for its content.

2 Tips and traps in buying software

After the initial layout for the computer itself, computer software is the next most expensive consideration. If the computer hardware world changes rapidly, the software world changes continuously. Every week brings new programs and updates of familiar ones. This chapter offers tips, traps and information about aspects of software buying.

Tip

Choose your wordprocessing package carefully. It is likely to be the one you use most.

It is widely acknowledged that wordprocessing accounts for the largest proportion of time given to personal computer work. Choose your own wordprocessing package with care. If you work in a hospital, clinic or college, you may have little choice over the type of wordprocessor you use: you may have to use the one on the network. If this is the case, it seems to be a reasonable idea to use the same wordprocessor at home (although you will have to buy your own copy).

At the time of writing, the three main *Windows* wordprocessing packages are *Word for Windows*, *WordPerfect for Windows* and *AmiPro*. There are, however, many others and very many DOS wordprocessors, of which *WordPerfect for DOS* still leads the market. However, wordprocessors are almost 'personal' things. One user's idea of an easy to use and comprehensive package is not necessarily someone else's.

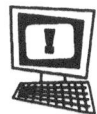

Trap

The price quoted by software manufacturers is not likely to reflect the real price.

For some strange reason, the manufacturer's quoted price for software rarely reflects the price that you can pay for it. The discrepancy between the one and the other is sometimes considerable. For example, in recent months, it has been possible to buy software that manufacturers quote as costing £399 for under £100. Some manufacturers, Microsoft being an example, have stopped quoting recommended prices in appreciation of this state of affairs. If you are reading advertisements published by the manufacturer, bear this in mind.

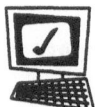

Tip

Consider buying software by mail order.

Some of the best bargains in software are to be found in the computer magazines. Such bargains cover all types of software – the big name products as well as the smaller, less known ones.

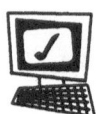

Tip

Computer magazines often give you working copies of software.

Many of the regular computer magazines are sold with a disk attached to the front cover – sometimes two disks. These often contain important shareware products and sometimes full versions of commercial programs. These versions are sometimes time-limited (you cannot use them after a certain date); others are cut-down versions of the programs that you can buy. Still others contain the whole, uncut program. If you are considering a range of different programs, these disks can help you to appreciate the 'look and feel' of a program and to try it out before you buy the full package.

  If you are working to a limited budget, look out for magazines that contain a whole, commercial program. These are often the 'version before the latest' of the program and represent extremely good value. After all, all you pay for is the magazine. Note, too, that many magazines give away further program disks with their subscription offers. These can also be a very good way of getting started with software.

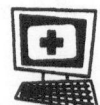

Help

A software buyer's checklist.

There is a variety of questions that you should ask about different sorts of software before you buy it. Stephens (1993) offers this useful and comprehensive list of questions. While not all of Stephens' lists will be used by every buyer, they offer a useful resource for the beginner as well as the more advanced buyer.

General

- Slick, consistent interface?
- Supports DDE and OLE where appropriate?
- Three-dimensional look and feel?
- Compatible with other software?
- On-line tutorial?
- Good technical support?
- Stable?
- Help system large enough to stop you constantly referring to the manual?

Wordprocessors

- Spell checker?
- Fully WYSIWYG ('What you see is what you get') in operation?
- Supports different file formats – can your old files be converted?
- Built-in graphical tools?
- Templates for envelopes and labels?
- Easy to perform a mailmerge?
- Easy macro language?
- Automatic index and table of contents?

Desktop publishing

- Handles spot and process colour?
- Automatic kerning?
- Support for large type sizes?
- Support for ATM and TrueType?
- Flows text between pages and columns and around graphics?
- Rotates objects?

- Automatic text effects like drop caps?
- Handles imported text and graphics from many different sources?

Databases

- Relational or flat-file?
- Stores pictures as well as text and numbers?
- Supports Query By Example?
- Easy mailmerge and form documents?
- Easy-to-learn programming language?
- Report generation?
- Transaction log?
- Forms designer for screen and output?

Spreadsheets

- Multidimensional?
- Three-dimensional graphics?
- Automatic formatting?
- Linked worksheets?
- What-if analysis?
- Easy annotation?
- Manual and automatic recalculation?

Drawing programs

- Handles both TrueType and Adobe Type Manager fonts?
- Generates colour separations for commercial printing?
- Bezier curves?
- Rotates and mirrors objects?
- Gradient fills?
- Different colour libraries?
- User-defined grid and drawing guides?
- Clip art?

Communications

- Automatically generated script language?
- Support for the most important file transfer protocols – X/Y/Z modem and Kermit?
- Emulation of common terminal types?
- Large dialling directory?
- Fax facility?
- Support for a range of modems?
- Keyboard remapping?
- Automatic redial when busy?

Development tools

- Creates true compiled programs or does it need a Visual Basic-style library?
- Comes with all the necessary *Windows* development tools, including a resource editor and the help compiler?
- Extensive on-line help?
- Visual environment?
- Creates DLLs as well as EXEs?
- Supports multimedia and pen computing?
- Compiler runs in the background?
- *Windows*-hosted debugger?

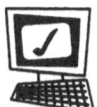

Tip

Listen to the experts but then go your own way.

People get used to the software that they use themselves. They then tend to think that the programs they use are the 'best' ones and this often leads them to recommend only those programs. Take advice from colleagues about what software they use, then choose from the range. It is also useful to read software reviews and to apply for demonstration disks that many companies supply.

Tip

Don't buy more software than you need.

It is sometimes tempting if you are setting up a department or buying for a research project to buy a wide range of different sorts of software just in case you need those programs. This can lead to the following problems:

- Too large a program is used for a relatively simple procedure.
- Other programs, such as wordprocessing programs (which now have a surprisingly large number of functions), are underused.
- Staff have to learn to use a range of programs instead of concentrating on a few well-chosen ones. This can increase the likelihood of errors.

It is probably best to buy software gradually and on an 'as you need it' basis. The exception to this is if you are buying a package of programs with your computer or a special offer – quite often advertised by manufacturers – of a range of programs packaged into one box. The latter can offer extremely good value for money.

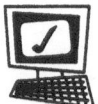

Tip

Buying the 'last but one' issue of a software program can be an economical way of acquiring software.

If budgets are limited, it is usually possible to buy a slightly earlier version of the program that you want. This means that you will be missing out on some of the very latest additions to the software but you will also save a considerable amount of money. Companies often sell off previous versions of programs at very much reduced prices. Look, too, for 'software sales' in which older versions are often included.

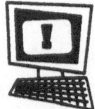

Trap

Remember that software is covered by copyright laws. You cannot usually use it on more than one machine.

Normally, you must not use a computer program on more than one machine (although see the next tip). The analogue that is sometimes used to explain the copyright law in this respect is that of a book. While you can read a book in various places and you can transport it, you may not copy it so that more than one copy of the copy you bought is circulating at any given time. Thus if you use a program at work you are legally bound not to copy it for home use. Nor are you free to share the program that you use at work with other colleagues in your office or department. Generally, every computer is required to have its own set of computer programs, bought for that machine and no other.

Tip

Some of the larger companies allow you to use one copy of their program at work and one at home, without buying two copies of the product.

Some enlightened companies, including WordPerfect, have introduced a more flexible approach to the use of their programs. They have suggested that the user may copy a program that is used at work for use at home – as long as the two copies are never used simultaneously. This means that if you use *WordPerfect for Windows* at work, you can make a copy for your notebook computer so that you can use it at home. What you cannot do is lend your notebook computer to a colleague so that both of you are using the program at the same time. All of this may seem rather pedantic but copyright rules in computing need protecting in the same way as they do in other forms of publishing. I wouldn't be too pleased if you made numerous copies of this book and distributed it to your friends – and neither would the publishers! So it is with computer software.

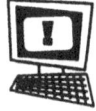

Trap

An upgrade in software becomes part of the original software package.

Software companies tend to publish new versions of their programs very frequently – sometimes as often as once or twice a year. This usually means that current users of the program can upgrade for a nominal sum. Note, however, that if you sell such software, you cannot sell it as two packages: the original program and the upgraded version. You have bought the upgrade on trust from the manufacturer and it is assumed, by all parties, that you really do own the original.

Tip

Register your software.

All software comes with a registration form. This gives the manufacturer proof that you are a *bona fide* user of the program. Registration
is usually a prerequisite of seeking help directly from the manufacturer.
If you ring a software company's user helpline, the first thing you will
be asked for is your registration number which will be checked against
their database of registered users. If you haven't registered, you are
unlikely to get help. Registration can also mean that you may be
entitled to free or reasonably priced upgrades to the program as they
are developed.

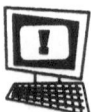

Trap

Often, you do not buy your software at all – even when you pay for it!

If you read the small print on the envelope containing software disks,
you will usually find that you have not bought the program but only
the right to use it. You will also note that when you open the envelope
you do so having agreed not to tamper with the software in any way
and not to copy it.

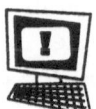

Trap

Help from software manufacturers is not always free.

Until recently, if you bought a program from a large software company,
you could rely on there being a free phone line for help with setting up
and running that program. In recent years, a number of companies
have started to charge for help and you may be asked to quote your
credit card number when ringing such helplines. Make sure that you
really do need help before you ring and pay for it.

Tip

Consider trying shareware.

Shareware is software that is sold on a try-before-you-buy basis. You
purchase a copy of the program that you need from a shareware
supplier for a nominal sum – the cost of copying the program, posting
it to you and a small profit margin. It is usual to pay between £3 and £5

for this service. You are then free to try out the program for between 30 and 60 days, depending on the contract. After that time, if you want to continue to use the program you are required to register your use with the author of the program and you pay a registration fee for this. Even taking into account registration, shareware is almost always a cheaper option than buying commercial software. Much of it is excellent and shareware should not be considered a second rate option.

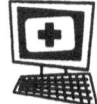

Examples of shareware programs.

Help

There is a wide range of shareware programs available, covering all the types of application that you can buy. A shortlist of the various sorts of programs includes.

- organizational programs;
- calculators;
- computer help programs;
- freeform database programs;
- full database managers;
- desktop publishing programs;
- specialist health care programs;
- spreadsheets;
- virus protection programs;
- wordprocessors;
- graphics programs;
- therapeutic and health related programs;
- computer utilities.

I have described many of these programs in *Personal Computing for Health Professionals*, also published by Chapman & Hall. Shareware is available in both DOS and *Windows* formats. Examples of shareware programs for *Windows* are described in Chapter 5.

Companies that supply shareware include:

The Public Domain and Shareware Library
Winscombe House
Beacon Road
Crowborough
East Sussex TN6 1UL

PCL Software Ltd
1 Silvey Grove
Spondon
Derby DE21 7GH

UK Euro Disk
5–11 Bull Street
West Bromwich
West Midlands B70 6EU

Testware UK Ltd
46 The Avenue
Harrogate
North Yorkshire HG1 4QD

SHS Shareware
19 Carshalton Road
Camberley
Surrey GU15 4AQ

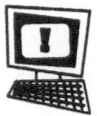

Trap

Shareware is not free.

You **must** register shareware if you continue to use it. The shareware system depends on trust and if the system is to continue then share-ware authors must be paid for their work. Registration usually brings you the latest version of the program, more extensive information about running the application and details of any new programs or upgrades.

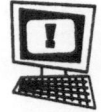

Trap

Shareware is not the same as public domain software.

Companies that handle shareware often offer public domain software too. Public domain programs are ones that the author has agreed can be used, free of charge, by other users. Once you have paid the shareware company the nominal fee for copying and sending you the program, you are free to use it and share it with others. However, shareware is not public domain software.

Tip

Consider using an integrated package.

Many of the larger software companies make **integrated** programs. These are sets of separate but linked applications. Usually, the integrated package includes a wordprocessor, a spreadsheet and a database program. Examples of these are *Works* (Lotus), *Works* (Microsoft) and *Window Works* (PFS).

Some of the larger companies also package together complete but separate programs (usually, a complete wordprocessor, spreadsheet and database) into one package. These differ from true, integrated packages in that they are 'stand alone' programs in their own right. They differ in the degree to which they interact with each other. Examples of these sorts of packages include *Office* (Microsoft), *Borland Office* (Borland) and *SmartSuite* (Lotus). These also represent excellent value for money and one of these packages is usually priced even more competitively that any single program contained within them.

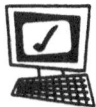

Tip

Draw up a list of the activities you are likely to carry out on your computer.

In order to find out what sorts of programs you need, consider the uses to which such programs will be put. Consider the following questions and answers:

- Do you need to produce letters, reports, essays, manuscripts or other mainly textual documents? You need a wordprocessing program.
- Do you need to add up columns of figures and keep large, numerical datasets on which you perform simple and complex calculations? You need a spreadsheet.
- Do you need to keep structured records of patients, clients, notes, appointments? You need a database program – increasingly called **database management software**.

- Do you need to draw charts and tables or prepare OHPs and other teaching and presentational aids? You need a graphics or presentations program.
- Do you need to keep track of appointments or plan management and research strategies? You need a personal information manager.
- Do you need to perform complicated statistical computations on large datasets? You need a statistics program.

Tip

Do you need anything more than a wordprocessor?

Despite the issues raised in the previous tip, it is important to appreciate that many of the larger wordprocessing packages can carry out many of the functions described above. *WordPerfect for Windows*, for example, has a built-in spreadsheet function and a graphics function. *Word for Windows* also has an extensive graphics section and an excellent built-in facility for developing charts and graphs. You may find that if you choose a fully featured wordprocessing program – particularly of the *Windows* variety – you won't need any other program for most of your work.

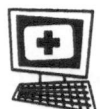

Help

Changing from DOS software to *Windows* software.

In a paper about changing from DOS to *Windows*, Waddilove (1992) suggests the following ten stages:

1. Hardware

First, to run *Windows* at all, you need a certain type of personal computer. The latest version of DOS calls for at least a 286 processor and you are likely to need between 3 and 4 megabytes of RAM to run it successfully. Also, the program occupies a large amount of hard disk space so an 80–100 megabyte hard disk is to be recommended.

2. Configuration

Before you install *Windows*, you need to make sure that your AUTOEXEC.BAT file does not contain pop-up programs (or 'terminate and stay resident' programs) that might conflict with the running of *Windows*.

3. Installation

The installation of *Windows* is usually fairly straightforward and the first disk of the program contains a simple 'setup' program that helps you to load automatically.

4. Fine tuning

Once *Windows* is loaded, you can check whether or not it will run with any disk-caching programs that you have. A disk-cache program helps other programs to run more quickly but some will work with *Windows* and some will not. After basic installation, you can check whether or not the ones that you have will work.

5. Customizing

Windows can be customized in various ways. Waddilove (1992) suggests at least the following options:

- altering the amount of space between the icons on the screen;
- modifying the width of the borders around the individual windows;
- changing the colour scheme and the 'wallpaper' that decorates the back of the screen;
- modifying the speed of the cursor movement when you use it with a mouse.

6. DOS programs

Windows usually checks to see what programs are on your hard disk as it is installing itself. When it finds a program, it incorporates its name into the icon system and offers you the chance to fire up the program from the program manager. Sometimes, though, DOS based programs are missed at installation. At this stage, you can manually install DOS programs so that each of them has its own icon.

7. Accessories

Various 'add-ons' are available to work alongside and with *Windows*. As you get more used to *Windows* you may want to try some of these as many are available as shareware (the concept of shareware is discussed in Chapter 8). Also, various accessories are packaged with *Windows*. You get a simple wordprocessor called *Write*, a notebook program, a clock and a calculator. You may want to spend time getting to know these accessories. They are also a useful means of learning about the total concept of *Windows*.

8. Windows programs

More and more programs are being written specifically for the *Windows* environment. For example, the well-known wordprocessors *WordPerfect* and *Word* have both been rewritten to run in *Windows* although both are also still available as DOS-only applications. Again, you may want to add these to your collection of programs. One of the strengths of the *Windows* environment is that many programs written for *Windows* share a common user interface. That is to say that the screen and menu layout are similar when you move between programs. Usually, the menu bar is at the top of the screen and once you have learned one *Windows* program, you will find subsequent ones easier to learn.

9. Utilities

One of the important utilities that is available for *Windows* is various font packages. The word **font** strictly refers to sets of print types. Increasingly, though, it is being used in a more general way to refer to 'typefaces'. For example, this book is printed in Palatino font. Add-on font programs are available from third party suppliers to add interest to what you see on the screen and what is printed out.

10. Deleting DOS programs

If you are finally sold on *Windows*, you may, as a final step, want to delete your DOS based programs altogether. My suggestion would be that if you do this, you hang on to the disks in case, at a later date, you decide to switch back. Whilst *Windows* is certainly more attractive as a user–computer interface, it is also much slower. At the time of writing, I have found it prudent to stick with DOS. By the time this book appears in print, it seems likely that I will have had to convert to *Windows* – simply because almost all manufacturers of software appear to be producing *Windows* based products at the expense of DOS based ones. Only a longer term appraisal of the product will enable users to decide whether or not *Windows* really is the ideal environment.

Tip

Learn *Windows* thoroughly.

Windows not only manages your programs and the way you work with those programs, it also sets the standards for the ways those programs operate. By learning all about *Windows* you are also learning all about a range of other programs.

Tip

Most *Windows* programs are organized in similar ways.

Although there are many advantages to using *Windows*, one of the key ones is that most *Windows* programs have similar user interfaces. This means that most *Windows* programs have a menu list at the top of the screen that is organized in the following groups:

File	Edit	View	Insert	Format	Tools	Window	Help

Clicking with the mouse on any one of these menu headings reveals a pull-down menu of other commands. This sort of uniformity amongst programs makes them very much easier to learn.

Tip

Use the *Windows* Print Manager with your *Windows* programs.

Almost all programs written to run under *Windows* can make use of the *Windows* Print Manager. This is an **applet** or small application within *Windows* that allows you to set a standard printer and font setting. When you print documents using the Print Manager, these standard settings are always used. Also, once a document is sent to the Print Manager, you are returned directly to your program and no further computing time is tied up with the printer. Using the Print Manager can help you to be more consistent in the way you print – despite using a range of different programs. It can also be quicker to print in this way than to use the program's own printer settings.

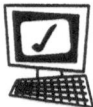

If you use only DOS programs, *Desqview* may be of more use to you than *Windows*.

Desqview is another program enabling you to multitask – to run more than one program at a time. *Desqview*, however, is for DOS rather than *Windows* programs although a combination of DOS, *Windows* and *Desqview* will run if you want it to. To run *Desqview 386*, you need a 386 or 486 computer and it is advisable to have more than 640K of RAM. There is, however, another version of *Desqview* for 286 computers.

The main *Desqview* program is both simple to install and easy to use. You install it onto your hard disk and, during installation, the program searches your hard disk for programs. From that search, *Desqview* automatically develops a menu system which includes those programs.

When you load *Desqview*, you are presented with that menu and from it, you start up the program that you need. When you want to switch to another program, you simply press ALT and back comes the menu. You are then free to load up your second (and third and subsequent) program(s), as required. Each program runs in a half-screen 'window' and you can switch between these windows (and, thus, between your programs) by tapping twice on the ALT key. If you don't like working in a window, you simply press ALT + Z and the current program fills the screen. When you next want to swap programs, pressing ALT takes you back to the menu.

Desqview offers you a simple-to-use way of working with a variety of programs and lets you switch between them in a few seconds. To work with large programs, quickly, you will need a fair amount of memory. If you do not have that memory, *Desqview* simply ships your programs out to disk and still lets you recall them but a little more slowly. Either way, you are saved the trouble of closing down one program simply to look at another. When you 'leave' a particular program, you are later 'returned' to exactly the spot that you left.

Make sure your computer's memory is correctly set up.

To make full use of *Windows* and *Desqview*, you need to make sure that those programs can access all of the RAM that you have available. There is a fuller discussion of memory issues in the next chapter. Here, suffice it to say that while *Windows* can 'find' all of the memory that is available, *Desqview* and other programs need to be 'shown' that memory is available. For this, you need a memory management program. Fortunately, one is supplied with DOS but it does need to be set up correctly.

Tip

Backup all your data files.

You must backup files as you go. This is the golden rule of computing. Whatever data files are on your hard disk should always exist as copies on floppy disks. Hard disks are much more reliable than they used to be but, as mechanical devices, they do and will fail. It is also possible, in extreme circumstances, for your hard disk to be corrupted in some way. I once tried to uncompress a compressed hard disk. The decompressing process didn't work and I lost all of the files on my hard disk. I didn't have backups of all my files and these were lost. **Always** do backups!

Tip

You do not normally need to backup all your program files.

The exception to the rule about backing up is program files. These are the files that run your programs and there may be many of them – particularly in a *Windows* application. It is not usually necessary to back these up to floppy disks or to a tape streamer as you already have copies of them as originals. However, there is a problem in this approach. If your hard disk does become corrupted and you needed to reinstall your programs, if you do not have floppy disk backups of them you will lose all the custom settings that you have developed while working with the program. Most people, as they learn more about their programs, like to change certain features. They develop shortcut keystrokes, macros, special layouts and templates. All of these are lost if you do not backup either the whole of a program's files or at least the file containing the changes you have made. You can usually find the name of the file that contains any customization in the manual accompanying your software. Since my own experience of a hard disk becoming corrupt, I have installed a tape streamer and I have a single tape containing everything on the hard disk. I do a complete backup of the whole hard disk at least once a fortnight and make incremental backups every times I use the computer. More tips about backup procedures are offered in Chapter 6.

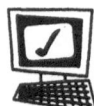

Tip

Read the manuals.

This may seem a rather obvious tip but many people do not read the manuals that are supplied with programs. This may be because some of the larger commercial programs come with multiple sets of manuals. Programs like *Paradox for Windows*, for example, come with four or five rather hefty manuals. However, nearly all good software also comes with a 'Getting Started' manual that tells you all you need to know to get up and running. After that, consult the manuals on an 'as you need to' basis. In the end, almost all of the information you need to use the program is in there somewhere. Given the fact that software companies are beginning to charge for telephone help, this sort of reading can save you money.

Cynical and vulgar computer journalists – probably out of impatience – have abbreviated the phrase Read the Manuals to RTFM.

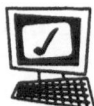

Tip

Some programs use special devices to protect their use.

Annoying, if understandable devices are used by some companies to make sure that only registered users have access to their programs. There are various levels of this sort of protection. Some companies insist that you ring them to be supplied with a code word or a number which you then type in at installation of the program. Without this word or number it will be impossible to make an installation. Other programs require that you always start the application from a special floppy disk that is inserted as you switch on the program. Finally, a few companies supply **dongles** with their software. These are devices that plug into the back of your computer and must be present if the program is to run.

Fortunately, most software companies trust the end user to pay for their products and most programs are not copy-protected in this way.

If you use a password, use the same one for all your files.

You may want to protect your files by attaching a password to them. This is particularly important if you use your computer for storing case notes or other text concerning patients or clients. If you do this, consider using the same password for all your files. If you begin to use multiple passwords, the likelihood of your forgetting one or more of them increases.

When choosing a password, bear in mind two things. First, make it one that you can remember easily – personalize it in some way. Second, make it a fairly unlikely mixture of numbers and letters. You might, for example, combine the first three digits of your birthdate with the first three letters of your sister's first name, reversed. Thus, if your date of birth is 14th July 1960 and your sister is called Jane, your password would 147naj.

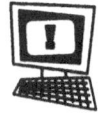

Some software and many networks can lock you out if you don't remember your password.

Learn your password well and type it in carefully. While almost all software and network systems allow you up to three tries at entering that password, some will then lock you out of the program or the system. This is an additional level of security. Be particularly careful if you set up a password to let yourself into the system when you turn it on. This, on the face of it, seems like a good idea. It means that no one can even get to the opening screen when the computer is turned on. Unfortunately, that 'no one' includes you! If you make a mistake in typing in your original password, you may inadvertently lock yourself out of your own computer.

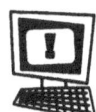

Don't use swearwords as passwords.

If you were attempting to 'crack' other people's passwords, what words would you try first? Chances are you would try swearwords or the person's name, street name or telephone number. For these reasons, when you devise a password, don't use these sorts of words or names.

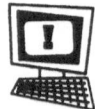

Trap

Don't forget your password.

The nature of software programming usually means that if you forget your password no one can access files. This includes the manufacturers of the software. Make sure that your password is committed to memory or that it is written down somewhere so that, if you forget it, you are not completely locked out of your files.

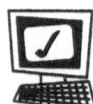

Tip

You can use passwords selectively.

If you are a senior clinician, a manager or an educator, you can adjust the levels of passwords that are used on a system. For example, if you organize a database of patients' or clients' names, addresses and clinical notes, you may be able to enter a password that makes the clinical notes available only to you. Or you can adjust the password system so that someone else can read the database but cannot make alterations to it. If you are working in a sensitive health care context you may find this selective password facility particularly useful.

Tip

Learn new software on a 'need to know' basis.

Don't try to learn everything about a new program at one sitting. Learn how to open the program, save a file and close the program. Look at the main menus and experiment a little. Then use the program. You can learn the more esoteric features as you need to use them.

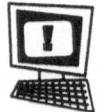

Trap

Make sure that you become aware of all features of a program.

This is the flip side of the above tip. While it is usually useful to learn about new programs on a 'need to know' basis, try also to learn all the features of that program over a period of time. It is not uncommon to find people using only about half of a program's features.

Tip

When you know one *Windows* program, you know the lot!

This is not the whole truth but it is not far off it. Because *Windows* programs use a common user interface, if you know one *Windows* program well, you are likely to find others very easy to use. Open any new *Windows* program and you will find a menu system at the top of the screen that you operate with the mouse. You will usually find, too, a button bar of some sort just below this menu system. The buttons give you access to many of the common functions of the program.

Tip

Have a break from a program and then go back to it.

This is an odd tip. I have found that if I learn a reasonable amount about a new program and then have a few weeks break from it I return to it and immediately learn a lot more about it. It is as though a break from the program helps in the learning process.

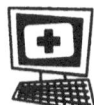

Help

There are a number of American health care related and other journals and newsletters that can help you decide on what software you need.

Here is a shortlist of some of the journals that are available. If they are not available in your library, it is worth considering borrowing some of them through the Inter-Library Loan scheme:

- *AI Expert*
- *AI Magazine*
- *AI Trends*
- *AI Week: The Artificial Intelligence Newsletter*
- *Assistive Technology*
- *Computational Medicine Technical Committee Newsletter*
- *Computer*
- *Computer News for Physicians*
- *Computer Talk: Directory of Medical Computer Systems*
- *Computer Use in Social Services Networks Newsletter*

- *Computerized Medical Imaging and Graphics*
- *Computers and Biomedical Research*
- *Computers and Medicine*
- *Computers in Biology and Medicine*
- *Computing in Healthcare*
- *Computers in Human Services*
- *Computers in Nursing*
- *Expert Systems: The International Journal of Knowledge Engineering*
- *Health Care Informatics*
- *Healthcare Financial Management*
- *International Journal of Clinical Monitoring and Computing*
- *Journal of Clinical Computing*
- *Journal of Computer Based Instruction*
- *Journal of Educational Computing Research*
- *Journal of Educational Technology Systems*
- *Journal of Medical Systems*
- *Knowledge in Society*
- *Methods of Information in Medicine*
- *National Report on Computing and Health*
- *Nurse Educators Microworld*
- *Physicians and Computers*

RECOMMENDED READING

Harvey, G. (1992) *Excel for Dummies*, IDG Books. Available from Computer Manuals, 50 James Road, Tyseley, Birmingham B11 2BA. Telephone: 021-706-1188

Excel is the bestselling spreadsheet package for running under *Windows*. Anyone who has to work with rows and columns of figures will soon find spreadsheets invaluable. They let you do all the usual arithmetical functions plus fairly complicated computations on large number sets. *Excel*, like *Windows* itself, allows you to work in a systematic way: if you can get around *Windows* you will soon get the hang of *Excel*.

If not, here is an excellent 'idiot's guide' to the program. Billed as 'a reference for the rest of us', the book is aimed at beginners. It is sometimes possible to imagine that 'beginners' means 'children' to the author of this book. The American, rather forced humour is sometimes a bit overwhelming, with chapters and subheadings such as 'Fancying Up the Figures' and the rather bizarrely named 'Just Put on a Happy Toolface'. The author is keen that you should adopt a fairly lighthearted approach to learning the program.

Once you get used to this lightheartedness, it has to be said that the book is an excellent introduction to *Excel*. It begins with a description of the program, takes you through the basics of setting up a spreadsheet and then, gradually, takes you into the more arcane aspects of the program. It closes with chapters of useful tips and tricks about how to make the program more usable (or, in the ugly language of the experts, 'increase its functionality') and a detailed glossary. The book also contains a 'cheat sheet' which is a guide to all the main keystrokes used in the program. American publishers really know how to produce high quality computer guides and this one is no exception. It is attractive to look at as well as easy to read.

3 Tips and traps in setting up your machine

It is one thing to buy a computer. It is another to get it running efficiently. Many people just take them out of the box, plug them in and starting running them. While you can do it this way – usually – if you want to get the best out of your computer it is better to spend a little time getting to know how to set it up optimally. This is especially true if you use *Windows* and *Windows* programs. There are all sorts of things you can do to make *Windows* run faster and more effectively. This chapter is about setting up your computer.

Tip

Take your time in getting your machine up and running.

Most people are keen to get their computers up and running once they have bought them. However, they usually come in a variety of packages containing the monitor, the keyboard, the main computer box and various cables and manuals. Before you do anything else, make sure that you have all the pieces of equipment that you should and read the first or introductory chapter of your first manual. It is usually about unpacking and setting up your computer. Follow the instructions carefully and do not assume that because you have set up hi-fi or television systems in the past, a computer system must be equally as straightforward. Usually it is, but you need to check that there are no special instructions relating to your computer that need to be observed before you switch on.

Tip

Make sure you send off your registration document.

Your registration document allows you to seek help from the manu-facturers and validates your warranty agreement. Complete this and send it off the day that you take delivery of your new computer.

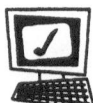

Tip

Leave the computer running for the first three days.

Most breakdowns in computers occur within the first 72 hours. Consider leaving your computer on, continuously, for the first three days. If it survives this period – and it probably will – it will normally run for very much longer periods without any problems. Some authori-ties suggest that you should leave your computer on indefinitely and that it is the switching on and off that causes the most strain on the system.

Tip

Dos and *Windows* should be preinstalled.

Previously, when you bought a computer, you usually had to install DOS and *Windows* (if it was supplied at all) before you ran any software. This is not normally the case today. Most computer companies preins-tall DOS and *Windows* prior to sending out new machines. Check that this is the case with your computer before reaching for the DOS or *Windows* disks.

Tip

Install DOS if you need to.

To install DOS, put the first disk into A: drive and type setup. Follow the on-screen instructions.

Tip

Install *Windows* if you need to.

To install *Windows* put the first disk into A: drive and type setup. Follow the on-screen instructions.

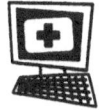

Help

Some key terms.

There are certain words and phrases that are used in the computing world that you need to get to know fairly quickly. Here is a shortlist:

DOS prompt. This is what you see on the screen once you have started up the computer and before you have started *Windows* or any other programs. The most basic form of the DOS prompt looks like this: C:\>

Applications. This is really another word for programs or the packages that you run on your computer. Thus your wordprocessor is an application or a program. So is your spreadsheet or database.

C prompt. Another term for the DOS prompt, except that it refers to the fact that you are in the root directory (see below).

Root directory. The main directory of the hard disk. The root directory is labelled 'C' and until you make 'subdirectories' it is the only place you have on your hard disk in which to store files.

Directories or subdirectories. These words are used interchangeably. They refer to sub 'containers' that you create within the root directory and in which you can store programs and data files. To use an office metaphor: if C: drive (or the root directory) is like a filing cabinet, then subdirectories are like the drawers within that filing cabinet. It is essential to learn how to create subdirectories. You must not store all your programs and data files in the root directory. This would be similar to putting all of your papers, reports and folders in a big cupboard – you would never be able to find anything quickly. Using subdirectories helps you to organize your files and programs. When you install programs onto your hard disk, they are automatically installed into their own subdirectories, created by the installation routine.

Tip

Check three files.

Ideally, the root directory should only contain three files: COMMAND.COM (which is an essential part of the running of your computer), CONFIG.SYS and AUTOEXEC.BAT (these two are described below). After that, all your other files should be stored in subdirectories. However, these three files **must** be in the root directory in order for your computer to start and to continue to work properly. Otherwise, keep your root directory 'clean'. This will help speed up your computing.

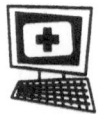

Help

What are the CONFIG.SYS and AUTOEXEC.BAT files?

These two files are essential to the smooth running of your computer. Robertson (1993) defines them as follows:

CONFIG.SYS. The main tasks of CONFIG.SYS are to set up the DOS internal system and to load external drivers from disk to create 'handles' to the hardware. It's read automatically, immediately after boot and can't alter the DOS setup at any other time.

AUTOEXEC.BAT. AUTOEXEC.BAT is a batch file, which runs commands and programs as if typed in at the command line. It can be run at any time from the DOS prompt as well as automatically after boot.

Tip

Get to know your CONFIG.SYS file.

You can view your CONFIG.SYS and AUTOEXEC.BAT files with a file manager. Two are included with DOS; they are called *Edlin* and *Editor*. Other, third party, file managers are also available.

A typical, optimized *Windows* and DOS CONFIG.SYS file will look like this:

```
DEVICE=C:\WINDOWS\HIMEM.sys
DOS=HIGH, UMB
COUNTRY=044,,C:\DOS\COUNTRY.SYS
FILES=40
BUFFERS=10
DEVICE=C:\WINDOWS\EMM386.EXE
STACKS=0,0
```

These lines are now briefly explained:

DEVICE=C:\WINDOWS\HIMEM.sys and DOS=HIGH, UMB
These commands allow most of DOS to be stored in the computer's
high memory.

COUNTRY=044,,C:\DOS\COUNTRY.SYS
This command makes sure that the date reads day/month/year.

FILES=40
BUFFERS=10
The **files** command dictates how many files can be opened at any one
time. Some of the larger programs automatically open many files at
once. A setting of 40 is a reasonable one for *Windows* programs.

The **buffers** command allows small amounts of data to be stored as
programs run and helps to speed up the running of your computer. If
you are using the SMARTDRV command in your AUTOEXEC.BAT file,
keep the value of this command low. Otherwise, set it at 40.

DEVICE=C:\WINDOWS\EMM386.EXE
This command allows the computer access to upper and expanded
memory.

STACKS=0,0
This is a command that has been 'left over' from earlier versions
of DOS. The default setting is STACKS=9,256 but a setting of
STACKS=0,0 usually works just as well and saves some memory.

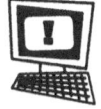

Trap

Learn more about handling your CONFIG.SYS file before you experiment.

CONFIG.SYS is essential to the running of your computer. Learn more
about it and always have a backup copy of it on a floppy disk before
you start experimenting with it.

If you do change your CONFIG.SYS file, change one line at a time
and then restart your computer. If you change lots of lines, it will
be more difficult to troubleshoot if things go wrong. Gradual and
incremental change is always the best approach with this file.

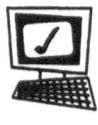

Get to know your AUTOEXEX.BAT file.

A typical, optimized, *Windows* and DOS AUTOEXEC.BAT file will look like this:

```
@ECHO OFF
C:\WINDOWS\MOUSE
C:\WINDOWS\SMARTDRV.EXE 1024 512
SET TEMP=C:\TEMP
PATH C:\DOS;C:\WINDOWS;
PROMPT $p$g
win
```

These lines are now briefly explained:

@ECHO OFF
This command tells the computer not to display this or the following lines when you start up the computer. This saves a lot of odd lines of text flashing by as you start up your machine.

C:\WINDOWS\MOUSE
This line installs the mouse.

C:\WINDOWS\SMARTDRV.EXE 1024 512
This command loads the disk-caching program *Smartdrive* which speeds up the running of your computer.

SET TEMP=C:\TEMP
This line makes sure that all your 'temporary' files created by *Windows* programs are stored in one central directory called TEMP. You must, of course, create a directory called TEMP in order for files to be directed there. To do this, at the DOS prompt, type the following: MD c:\temp.

PATH C:\DOS;C:\WINDOWS;
This command tells your computer where to look for files. If you have subdirectories included in this list (e.g. DOS, WINDOWS), you no longer have to type the whole of the path command to start up a program. Thus, with WINDOWS in the path, you can start *Windows* by typing 'WIN' at the DOS prompt, instead of moving to the *Windows* subdirectory first.

PROMPT pg

This command dictates what will show up on the screen at the DOS prompt. The format shown here will not only display 'C:\>' as the DOS prompt. Instead it will display that plus the name of the directory that is current. Thus, if you are in the *Windows* directory, you will see: 'C:\WINDOWS>'.

WIN

This final command, will fire up *Windows* every time the computer is switched on.

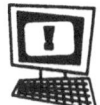

Trap

Learn more about handling your AUTOEXEC.BAT file before you experiment.

AUTOEXEC.BAT is essential to the running of your computer. Learn more about it and always have a backup copy of it on a floppy disk before you start experimenting with it.

If you do change your AUTOEXEC.BAT file, change one line at a time and then restart your computer. If you change lots of lines, it will be more difficult to troubleshoot if things go wrong. Gradual and incremental change is always the best approach with this file.

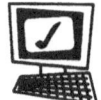

Tip

Make an emergency start-up disk.

This is vital. At some point, your hard disk will fail or you will make an error in editing your CONFIG.SYS file. If either of these things happens, the chances are that you will not be able to start your computer by merely switching it on. What you need is an emergency start-up disk that allows you to start the computer from A: drive.

First, format a new floppy disk with the command: A:\Format/s. The /s at the end of the command puts essential systems files onto the floppy disk. Then, copy over your AUTOEXEC.BAT, CONFIG.SYS and COMMAND.COM files to the floppy from your hard disk (they are in the root directory).

Label this disk clearly and do not use it for anything else. If your computer fails to 'boot up' from the hard disk, simply put the emergency disk in A: drive and restart your computer. The computer

Extended memory	All memory above 1 Mb
Upper memory	640 K – 1 Mb
Conventional memory	0 K – 640 K

Figure 3.1 Tyes of memory.

should start directly from the floppy disk and will allow you to access all your programs and files on C: drive. Once you have started your computer in this way, either edit your CONFIG.SYS or AUTOEXEC.BAT files or seek help from a computer expert as to what has caused the boot failure.

Tip

Check your mouse.

If your mouse fails to work properly, Venditto (1992) suggests the following:

1. If the mouse uses a roller, make sure it is rolling on a surface that provides adequate friction. The inexpensive mouse pads sold in computer stores can usually fix this problem.
2. If the mouse uses a roller, the interior may be dirty. You can usually pop open the plastic case that holds the rubber ball and clean out the interior, following the instructions in the manual.

3. Optical mice don't have rollers and work only when slid across the tablet or grid they came with. Contact the manufacturer of the mouse for assistance.

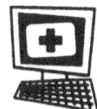

Help

Understanding memory.

All computers are supplied with RAM or random access memory. This is where programs and data files are 'stored' while they are being worked with on the computer. As soon as you switch the computer off, anything stored in memory is lost. There are three main sorts of memory: **conventional** memory, **upper** memory and **extended** memory and these are illustrated in Figure 3.1. There is another sort of memory called **expanded** memory which is in some ways an 'artificial' memory: the computer has to be properly set up to use expanded memory and only certain DOS programs need it. All *Windows* programs run in the other three sorts of memory.

The important thing to know about memory is that the computer that is not customized in any way cannot use any memory apart from conventional memory. If you have memory above 640K, you must use a **memory manager** to make sure that the computer and its programs can access it. You can have a computer with 4–8Mb but if it is not properly set up, all you have access to is the first 640K. DOS, as we shall see, comes with its own memory manager but this does not set itself up automatically. You must 'tell' the memory manager to work and this is explained in a later tip.

The exception to the above comments is the use of *Windows* which automatically accesses available extended memory. Even with *Windows* running, however, it is useful to use a memory manager as these free all-important conventional memory for use by DOS programs.

Tip

Consider third party memory managers.

Not every one can or wants to buy the latest computer. While 386 and 486 PCs are common now in many health care settings, individuals are likely to run lower powered 286 machines. These computers are ideal if your main computing needs involve word processing or the use of simple database programs. They are also an excellent bargain. Many companies now sell 286 computers at extremely low prices. This means that students, managers and teachers can nearly all afford a PC.

There are limitations, however. Less powerful computers mean that the most needs to be made of the equipment available. This is where two important products, *Qram* and *Desqview* come into their own.

The oddly named *Qram* is a memory manager. It helps the 286 to make best use of the computers available memory. If, for example, you have a computer that has 1 megabyte of RAM, you can only make use of the first 640K of memory without a memory manager of some sort. A memory manager is supplied with the operating system that comes with the computer but *Qram* is a much more sophisticated one. It analyses all of the available memory and then 'packs' the programs that are to be used into that memory in the most economical way. If, for instance, you use a pop-up database program in which you store your bibliographical references and you run this program 'over the top' of your wordprocessing program, then *Qram* will load the pop-up program in high memory. This leaves you much more conventional memory to use for your regular programs.

Qram is very easy to install from a single disk. An installation routine loads the program onto your hard disk. A companion program, *Optimize*, supplied with *Qram* offers yet another level of memory analysis and makes fine adjustments to memory to suit the particular requirements of your setup. Finally, a third program supplied with the package – *Manifest* – helps you to see how your memory is organized.

Set up your computer to use memory efficiently.

DOS6.0 comes with its own memory manager. At the C: prompt, type memmaker and the memory manager starts to do its work. You can choose from an **express** routine or a **custom** one. Choose express if you are not sure how you want to configure your computer's memory and the program will make all the decisions for you.

Tip

If you plan only to use *Windows* programs, you don't need expanded memory.

Most memory managers, including *Memmaker* (supplied with DOS), ask you if you require expanded memory. Many DOS programs make use

Tip

of expanded memory and if you use, for example, a DOS database program, you should allow the memory manager to configure some of your memory as expanded. *Windows* does not use expanded memory (although it will use all the extended memory that you can supply) and you can safely and usefully answer 'no' to the question about expanded memory when you use your memory manager.

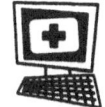

Help

Golden rules for working with a personal computer.

By way of a short reprise and as a means of summarizing many of the points in this book at the half-way mark, here are some golden rules that you **must** follow if you use a computer on a regular basis:

- Do backups. This is the first and last rule of all computing. You **must** backup files that are on your hard disk. Hard disks fail. You can corrupt your CONFIG.SYS and AUTOEXEC.BAT files. You can have power cuts that corrupt files. Be ready for any of these things. Make sure that, at any given time, you can always replace all of the files that are currently on your hard disk.

- Read the manuals. Although most computer software and hardware manuals wouldn't qualify for the opening rounds of the Booker Prize, they usually contain all the information you need to work with the programs or equipment you have bought. Use the reference manuals and use the indexes of those manuals. Most of your problems can be solved by taking a few deep breaths and delving into the manuals.

- If all else fails, use the helplines. Almost all software companies offer a hotline service for help. It is a sad fact that many now charge for this service. Have a number of things ready before you phone for help. First, you must have your registration number with you when you phone. No hotline will help you if you cannot quote the registration number. Second, try to make the call from your computer desk. It is always much easier if the person at the end of the phone can talk you through your problem. Third, have your credit card ready. You will be asked for your credit card number and the expiry date if the hotline is one that charges for the service.

- Learn more about your software. In quiet moments, try out some of the apparently more arcane features of your programs. Most people only use a very small percentage of a program's overall features. Wordprocessors in particular often have features that would be useful to very many people if only they knew about them.

- Learn hard disk hygiene. Hard disks and programs run much more efficiently if you take care of your hard disk. Here are some basic rules:
  1. Erase unnecessary files. Don't let your hard disk get full up with files that you never use.
  2. Defragment your hard disk regularly. There are a number of programs available to do this (DOS includes one called *Defrag*). Use such a program regularly to make sure that bits of your files are not spread all over the hard disk.
  3. Make regular total backups of the hard disk (if you have a tape streamer) or total backups of all your data files if you use floppies.
  4. Run Chkdsk (included with DOS) to check for any hard disk errors. Typing Chkdsk at the C: prompt will check the whole of your hard disk for 'lost clusters'. This is not the place to go into what these are; suffice it to say that you should check for them regularly. If you find any, it is usually safe to erase them. If you often find them, talk to a computer expert. He or she will probably want to see how you use your computer. There are a number of simple computing errors that can lead to lost clusters.

- Look after your health. This might seem an unnecessary injunction in a book for health professionals but I doubt that it is. Make sure that you don't sit at the computer for lengthy periods. Every ten minutes or so, do something different. Stand up, stretch, look away from the monitor for a little while. It is good practice not to arrange your computing facilities so that you don't have to get up. Getting up to feed paper into the printer – or even to switch a button on the printer – can be useful ways of breaking your rhythm. One of the biggest problems of computer use is that it encourages you to remain in one position for such a long time. Make sure that you move on a regular basis. If it helps, get a keyboard wrist-rest.

  Make sure that your seating and desk arrangements comply with European standards. There are strict regulations laid down about the type of equipment that should be made available to computer users in organizations. Make sure that you are familiar

with them. If you require one, ask for a footrest – your organization is obliged to supply you with one if you consider you need
it.

RECOMMENDED READING

Konicki, S. (1983) *Killer PC Utilities*, Que Corporation. Available from
Computer Manuals, 50 James Road, Tyseley, Birmingham B11 2BA.
Telephone: 021-706-1188

This is a huge paperback book containing very detailed information
about how to get the most out of your PC. It covers 'turbocharging'
your computer, understanding and maintaining the system, diagnosing
and troubleshooting and data recovery. This book takes you well
beyond the average computer manual and offers technical advice in a
straightforward and easy-to-follow format. Everything is here, from
inserting more memory chips to fitting a new hard disk and from
understanding DOS error messages to understanding computer viruses.
The book also comes with a disk containing a range of useful PC
utilities, including a disk spooler which will speed up printing, a screen
saver to prevent 'burn in' of your screen, a hard disk testing program
and a virus checking program. If you are serious about developing your
personal computing knowledge and want to know how to get to grips
with what's 'under the bonnet', this is the ideal reference book.

Goodman, J.M. (1993) *Hard Disk Secrets*, IDG Books. Available from
Computer Manuals, 50 James Road, Tyseley, Birmingham B11 2BA.
Telephone: 021-706-1188

This is billed on the front cover as 'Another Bestselling SECRETS book'.
How do they know this at first printing? On the other hand, you can
see why this is a bestseller. It is an authoritative treatise on almost all
aspects of hard disks. The first part is going to be of most use to the
general reader. It contains chapters on how hard disks work, how they
manage data, what to do when things go wrong and how to fit new
ones. The author even includes last-ditch emergency surgery for a
dying hard disk – apparently you hit it with a hammer to force it to
restart! Not for the fainthearted.

This is not just a book for beginners. Anyone who wants to build a personal computer and make the right purchasing choices will be well advised to read this. It contains a considerable amount of technical detail and it will be helpful for the person who buys a secondhand or 'job lot' hard disk. There is a considerable amount here on setting up and optimizing the hard disk.

The second section is all about *SpinRite* – a commercially available program for optimizing hard disks. I thought this was a bit naughty. Presumably you buy this book to find out all about hard disks and not necessarily to find out about *SpinRite*. However, more than 100 pages are given over to aspects of the program.

That aside, the book is clearly and authoritatively written and comes with the now almost obligatory floppy disk full of software utilities – some useful and some less so. There are no less than three 'head parking' programs on the disk. Strange, when you consider that most hard disks these days are 'self-parking'.

4 Tips and traps in using DOS

DOS or the disk operating system is the system you encounter every time you turn on your personal computer (unless, of course, you are using another sort of operating system but that is beyond the remit of this book). DOS is the 'framework' in which all your other programs run – including *Windows*. A little time spent in getting to know DOS is time well spent.

Tip

Check which version of DOS you are using.

If you are not sure which version you are running, type VER at the DOS prompt and the version number will be printed on the screen. This is useful if you are working with a program that only works with certain versions of DOS and if you are about to use that program on a computer that you are not familiar with.

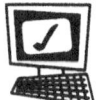

Tip

DOS is supplied with an excellent diagnostic program.

If you move to the DOS directory and type MSD you will start the *MS Diagnostics* program which will give you detailed information about:

- your computer;
- memory;
- printer ports;
- AUTOEXEC.BAT;
- CONFIG.SYS;
- many more facets of your computer and the way it is set up.

Tip

Installing a new version of DOS.

When you buy a new version of DOS you are supplied with about four or five compressed floppy disks. Simply insert the first one, move to A: drive and type Setup. This will allow you to install your new version of DOS over the old one. Respond to any questions on the screen. Most versions of DOS have an express setup routine and a custom routine. If you are in doubt about what your current needs are, use the express setup and then most of the installation decisions are made for you.

Tip

You can use *DoubleSpace* to 'double' your hard disk size.

From version 6.0, the disk compression program *DoubleSpace* was included as part of DOS. Simply typing DBLSPACE at the DOS prompt will fire up the program that can increase the space on your hard disk by nearly 50%. While there have been some problems associated with *DoubleSpace* described in the computing press, many people have used it with no problems at all. The important thing is to follow the on-screen instructions to the letter and to make sure that you are familiar with the section of the manual that covers *DoubleSpace*.

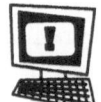

Trap

The *DoubleSpace* process cannot easily be reversed.

Consider the *DoubleSpace* process as permanent. While it is possible to 'un-DoubleSpace' a compressed hard disk, the process is not easy and it is not documented in the DOS manual. Make sure you know what you are doing and that you really do want to use disk compression before you start the process.

Tip

Consider compressing only part of your hard disk.

If you use the custom option when you run the *DoubleSpace* program, you can elect to compress only the empty part of your disk. This means that all the files that are on your disk already remain uncompressed. Only the empty section of the hard disk is compressed. This is the 'cautious' option for the person who is not sure that they trust disk compression.

You may want to consider a third party disk compression program.

Despite the fact that *DoubleSpace* is supplied with DOS, as we have seen, use of that compression program is fairly final. Some other third party compression programs allow you to 'decompress' should you need to.

Stacker (Stac) makes that possible. In fact, *Stacker* has become so well known that it is now common to hear of 'stacked drives' – the computer world seems to have adopted *Stacker* as something of a standard. And that comes as no surprise when you use the program.

This new version of the program is particularly useful in that it runs directly under *Windows* and is made to work with DOS 6.0. Now DOS 6.0 comes with its own, inbuilt hard disk compressor *DoubleSpace* but more of that in a moment.

Stacker is simple to set up. You put one of two disks in your floppy disk drive and follow the instructions on the screen. You can use the express setup to compress the whole of your hard disk or (if you are new to the program) the custom setup if you want to compress a number of disks. The program investigates your hard disk, compresses it and then optimizes the result through the use of a subset of the Norton defragmentation program. I found it took just under one hour to complete the compressing and setting up of a 120 megabyte hard disk which was three quarters full. I ended up with a new free disk space of 140 megabytes.

On first rebooting the computer, *Stacker* offers you the chance to install the *Stackometer* – a series of monitoring programs that run under Windows. These are very neatly realized. A 'speedometer' tells you how much free disk space is available and another section shows you the degree to which your hard disk has or has not become fragmented. Fragmentation occurs over time. As files are deleted from the hard disk and new ones written to it, sections of files and programs get deposited all over the hard disk. This happens whether or not you use *Stacker*. This sort of fragmentation slows down the running of your computer and it is in your interest to defragment it on a regular basis. Built into the *Stacker* suite of programs is its own defragmenter and the *Stackometer* will let you know whether or not you need to use it. This sort of feature would be useful on any computer – with or without a disk doubling program. For the compulsive tinkerer, there are all sorts of fine-tuning devices. Most people, I suspect, will be happy enough with the default settings.

Stacker works with a wide range of caching programs – programs that help to speed up your computer as it reads from and writes to the hard disk – and it will compress most sorts of hard disks, large or small, permanent or removable. It also runs with all of the standard high memory managers.

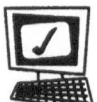

Tip

Use *Edit* to make adjustments to your CONFIG.SYS and AUTOEXEC.BAT files.

DOS contains two built-in text editors that will enable you to make adjustments to your CONFIG.SYS and AUTOEXEC.BAT files. There is an older and more complicated one called *Edlin* included in the DOS directory and one that is much easier to use, called *Edit*. *Edit* is started by moving to the DOS directory and typing *Edit* at the C prompt.

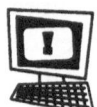

Trap

Edit needs QBasic in order to run.

Edit relies on the existence of the programming language supplied with DOS, called QBasic. The main QBasic file – QBASIC.EXE – must be present in the DOS directory in order for you to start up the *Edit* text editor.

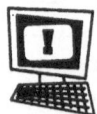

Trap

Always make backups of CONFIG.SYS and AUTOEXEC.BAT before you make adjustments.

CONFIG.SYS and AUTOEXEC.BAT files are essential for the correct starting of your computer. Before you make any changes to them, make sure that you have backups of both of these files on floppy disks. Then, if you make a mistake in your modifications, you can always restart the computer from your floppy. If you do not make backups, you are stuck. You can no longer start the computer from your DOS disks (from version 6.0 onwards) as the files on those disks are compressed. You must have backup copies of these two files.

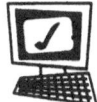

Tip

Third party text editors are sometimes easier to use.

Edlin is a complicated text editor to use. It remains as part of the DOS package because people who used earlier versions of DOS got used to using it. *Edit* is less complicated but you may still want to use a simple editor supplied by a third party company. There are various simple-to-use shareware text editor programs (e.g. *Boxer* and *QEdit*). There are also commercially produced text editors and one of the best is included in the WordPerfect Corporation's utilities package *Office*.

Tip

You can use your wordprocessor to make changes to CONFIG.SYS and AUTOEXEC.BAT.

You don't have to use a text editor to make changes to these files, you can use your wordprocessing program. Be careful, though. These two files must be saved in ASCII format and not as wordprocessing files. Most modern wordprocessors can save files in ASCII format and if you are sure you can remember to save them in this way, you should have no problems with this sort of editing. Before you make any changes to these two files you must make backups of them. Remember, your computer won't run properly without them. If you accidentally save these files as ordinary wordprocessing files, they will not work. They must be saved as ASCII files. For this reason and to avoid making mistakes, I find it easier to use a plain text editor to make changes to the files.

Tip

DOS commands are not 'case sensitive'.

You can type in DOS commands either in upper or lower case (capitals or small letters) or a mixture of both.

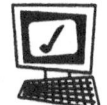

Tip

You can fastformat old floppy disks.

Usually, formatting disks with the DOS FORMAT command takes a little while. If you want to reformat an old disk so that you can put new files on it, you can use the fast format command. Put the used disk into drive A. Then use the command FORMAT a: /q /u for an 'instant' format.

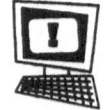

If you fast format a disk, you will not be able to 'unformat' the floppy.

If you use this method of formatting a used disk, you will not be able to use the UNDELETE command on the disk at a later date to 'rescue' files that were previously on the disk. The fast formatting command makes retrieval of old files impossible.

Six ways to launch DOS applications from within *Windows*.

Many health professionals will use DOS and *Windows* together. Edelhart (1992) identifies the following six ways to launch DOS applications from within *Windows*:

1. Add an icon to launch your DOS application from the Program Manager. Select *new* from the Program Manager file menu, specify that you're creating a program item, supply the name you want to appear with the icon and indicate the path and command you would normally use to execute the program.

2. Use the File Manager to launch a DOS program by locating the subdirectory containing its executable file and double-clicking on the filename entry.

3. If the program has a PIF file – either one you've created or one that *Windows* put together during setup – locate it and double-click on the PIF's name in the File Manager.

4. Use the Run command on the file menu in the Program Manager. When prompted for the name of the program you want to use, type the name of your application's executable file (including its path) or the name of the PIF that launches it and then press Enter.

5. Select the DOS prompt icon in the Program Manager to get to the DOS command line and then launch your application with the same commands you'd use outside *Windows*.

6. Or, finally, use third-party alternatives to the Program Manager, such as HDC's *Power Launcher* or Norton *Desktop for Windows*.

RECOMMENDED READING

Gookin, D. (1993) *The Microsoft Guide to Managing Memory with MS-DOS 6*, 2nd edn, Microsoft Press. Available from Computer Manuals, 50 James Road, Tyseley, Birmingham B11 2BA. Telephone: 021-706-1188

Computer memory is not the easiest thing to understand. Most books about computing contain a section on it and tell you the differences between conventional, extended and expanded memory. Whether or not this information is useful to you usually depends on the way in which the topics are described. Gookin's book does much more than offer a description: it offers direct and practical advice about all aspects of memory management. DOS 6 offers much more than previous versions. For a start, it offers disk compression and a memory manager of its own – *Memmaker*. Gookin covers these matters and much, much more.

The book begins with what appears to be a standard description of the different types of memory. What it is, however, is an intelligible description. Gookin's description made me understand, after some years, exactly what expanded memory is and why *Windows* doesn't need it. The book goes on to consider how your computer uses memory and how to add further RAM to your system and why you might want to do that.

There is a very useful chapter on the use of RAM disks and another on preparing your memory for using *Windows*. Like Gookin's other book *Optimizing Windows*, this one is clearly written and has all the hallmarks of Gookin's light and humorous touch. He has a gift for making the complex apparently simple. This book offers extremely good value for money and will be useful to any PC user.

Jamsa, K. (1992) *Jamsa's 1001 DOS and PC Tips*, Osborne/McGraw-Hill and Jamsa, K. (1993) *Jamsa's 1001 Windows Tips*, Jamsa Press. Available from Computer Manuals, 50 James Road, Tyseley, Birmingham B11 2BA. Telephone: 021-706-1188

Kris Jamsa undertook a courageous enterprise when he set out to find 1001 tips for the world's most frequently used operating system and then another 1001 tips for *Windows*. There must have been times when he wished he had aimed at 500 or, perhaps, 250. Generally, we should be grateful that he continued with his work. These two books contain more information than most casual users are likely to need and almost all the information that the regular user will.

The DOS book is the most successful. There is remarkably little padding here and huge numbers of really useful tips about setting up and using the DOS operating system. You can tell that Jamsa is a real computer expert. Many of the tips involve specially written batch files that can temporarily change the way in which your computer works. With the book comes a disk containing all of these batch files. Thus, if you are taken by a particular tip and note that it involves writing a special DOS command, you simply call up the appropriate batch file from the disk and the writing is done for you.

The 1001 tips are divided up into chapters. There are chapters about the computer system, managing memory, the keyboard and disks and managing files and directories. There is a series of contents pages which list all of the tips and an excellent index to help you find the ones that you want.

This is as much a book to dip into and to keep as a reference book as one to read through. You couldn't take in this much information at one sitting and, after all, the book is very large (I estimate about 600 pages although, oddly, the pages are not numbered). Also, there is some padding, to make up the 1001 tips. Empathic health care professionals will love the tip 'Understanding Your Keyboard Cable', for instance. And 'Push in the Turbo Button' may seem a little like page-filling. On the other band, you couldn't avoid learning a lot from this book, whether you are a complete beginner or a dyed-in-the-wool computer bore.

Obviously, *1001 DOS and PC Tips* has sold well. So much so that Jamsa formed his own company for the next book (modestly called the Jamsa Press). This is almost identical in layout and concept and, once again, offers a lot that is useful about getting around and using *Windows*. However, in this one there is a lot of padding. The early chapters, for example, offer details of how to set up the *Windows* environment and much of it repeats what is already in the *Windows* manual. Sometimes, too, the 'tips' format of the book gets a bit cumbersome. It would have been good, occasionally, to read a few paragraphs about a particular topic. Sometimes the page-filling is annoying. Tip 45, for example, is 'What is the File Manager.' Surely, anyone who uses *Windows* for more than ten minutes gets to realize that files are managed by a section of the program called the File Manager. This book, then, may have been better in a *500 Tips* format, for some are very useful.

This book covers not only basic *Windows* functions but DOS 6 and *Windows for Workgroups.* Anyone who has responsibility for managing a range of computers or a network will appreciate the information contained in these sections.

As with the DOS book, this one comes with a disk, very different to the one that accompanies the DOS book but just as useful. It contains, in compressed form, a program that allows you to look up the tips contained in the book. This is an excellent idea and one that I hope other computer writers will adopt. It means that you can have on-line help about almost all aspects of *Windows* and DOS at the touch of a couple of buttons or of the mouse. The program is like all *Windows* help programs and allows you to do searches, save sections of text, insert 'bookmarks' and print out sections of the help screens.

5 Tips and traps in using *Windows*

Windows has become just about the most widely used framework for organizing and running the PC. This chapter offers tips and traps about all aspects of *Windows* computing. Purists should note that '*Windows*' is singular. You say, for example, 'This computer has *Windows* on it and I use it'.

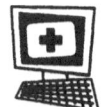

Help

What is *Windows*?

Windows is a program developed and produced by Microsoft that has to be loaded from the DOS prompt like any other. It does not replace DOS and you cannot run it on a machine that does not have DOS installed on it. Nicholson (1993) offers the following description of *Windows* essentials. *Windows*:

- provides a memory structure in which you can run both *Windows* and DOS applications;
- provides a multitasking mechanism that allows more than one program to run at any one time;
- provides an interface so that you can control the system;
- manages the links between your applications and the keyboard, mouse, display, printer, modem and so on;
- provides a mechanism that allows one application to interact with another.

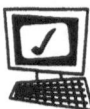

There is a built-in tutorial supplied with *Windows*.

To run the tutorial, perform the following steps.

Tip
1. From the Program Manager, select the Help menu.
2. Choose the *Windows* tutorial option. *Windows* will then start the tutorial. You can press Esc (Escape) any time that you want to leave the tutorial.

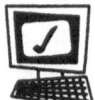

Be clear about what a 'window' is.

Windows is the program and a 'window' is a boxlike structure on the screen that can contain various things. A window can, for instance, contain a series of icons that allow you to start up programs. When you click on an icon you start up a program and this is displayed in another 'window'. You can have various 'windows' open on the screen at any given time and switch between them. When you run various programs in various windows, this is known as **multitasking**.

Tip

Switch quickly between open windows.

Imagine that you have your wordprocessor open in a window and you want to return to the Program Manager. All you have to do is to hold down ALT and press the TAB button on the keyboard. If you have various windows open, you can 'cycle' through them by continuing to press the TAB button while holding down the ALT button

Tip

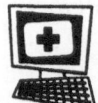

Become familiar with key features of *Windows*.

There are certain features that you must know about in order to work with *Windows* successfully. Table 5.1 highlights the names and functions of the main components of *Windows*.

Help

Table 5.1

Name	Function
Program Manager	The main window that contains all the main menus and program icon groups
Control menu box	Opens a window's control menu which lets you move, change the size of or close a window
Icons	Small, graphical representations of minimized windows of programs. Normally, if you double click on an icon, a program opens
Desktop	The background area behind all of the open windows (including the Program Manager)
Menu bar	The small horizontal section beneath the title bar which contains various menu names
Mouse pointer or cursor	The movable white arrow that can be moved across the screen by the mouse. This changes to an hour glass when *Windows* is busy performing a function and indicates that you have to wait
Title bar	The horizontal, narrow region right at the top of a window which usually contains the name of the program or document that you are working in. If you are in the Program Manager, this will contain the words 'Program Manager'
Minimize button	A small box at the top right hand corner of the screen which allows you to shrink an open window to an icon
Maximize button	A small box at the top right hand corner of the screen which allows you to increase the size of an open window
Border	Four edges that define and contain an open window
Workspace	The white area inside a window

Tip

Some software sticks to the *Windows* rules.

When Microsoft developed *Windows*, they laid down some conventions for programming software for *Windows*. Stephens (1993) identifies the issues that mark out programs that play by the rules. Look out for them in the *Windows* software that you choose. Programs that follow these rules are likely to be easier to learn that ones that break them.

Stephens suggests that programs that stick to *Windows* rules:

- have a tool bar for commonly used functions;
- have a status bar for information purposes;
- have a proper *Windows* help system;
- make use of the *Windows* common dialogues;
- provide a real WYSIWYG preview for printing;
- have the new three-dimensional look and feel;
- give you the maximum working area with the minimum of clutter;
- use scroll bars properly and have resizable windows;
- allow you to configure the colours and fonts they use;
- make best use of colour, particularly when displayed on a note-book's LCD screen.

Tip

Get used to the notion of an 'object' in *Windows*.

In lay terms, an 'object' in *Windows* is a single unit – a table, a chart, a picture or a special graphical item – that contains information. For example, in a *Windows* database, the table that contains your information is an object. So is the form in which you enter your information and the report form that allows you to present your information for printing out.

The point about objects is that they can be customized to a considerable degree, often through the use of the right hand mouse button. Often, if the cursor is 'inside' an object, you can click on the right mouse button and produce a menu that will allow you to change all sorts of features of that object: the font size, the colour, the shape of the object and so on. Just getting the hang of the idea of an object can help you to work with *Windows* programs very easily and in very flexible ways.

One of the programs that makes very considerable use of objects is the personal information manager *PackRat* (Polaris Software). At first glance, *PackRat* seems to be a very complicated program. Once you have mastered the idea of an object, however, it becomes very easy to use and very easy to customize to your own way of working. The same can be said of the database program *Paradox for Windows* (Borland).

You don't have to use the Program Manager shell.

Although *Windows* comes with its own start-up user screen, known as the Program Manager, not everyone finds this particularly useful or comprehensive enough. While the Program Manager will allow you to fire up your programs and group program icons together, it does little more than that. You may prefer to use a third-party replacement for it.

There are at least two options here. One is to use a complete replacement 'shell'. *PC-Tools for Windows* (Central Point Software) offers a comprehensive example of this sort of replacement. Alongside the other 'tools' (described in Chapter 6), *PC-Tools* offers a comprehensive screen management program. It offers a series of 'desktop' layouts that can be customized by the user. You may, for instance, have a different 'desktop' for each of your projects. You might have one that organizes your research projects, another that groups together all the programs and files that relate to patients or clients and another that is tied to 'personal' applications. Although this program offers a huge amount of flexibility and customization to the 'power' user, the newcomer may find it a bit daunting.

The other option is to use a 'minimalist' type of program and utility program. *Dashboard* (Hewlett Packard) is an excellent example of this approach to Program Manager replacement. *Dashboard* uses the analogy of the car dashboard. You are offered a slim bar on the screen which you configure to contain miniature program icons (for firing up your programs), a 'speedo' which dynamically monitors your memory usage, a printer manager and a method of switching between any programs that are currently open. The 'dashboard' is almost infinitely customizable. The real minimalist can reduce it to a single row of program icons which always sits at the bottom or down the side of the screen. A single click on any icon is sufficient to start up the program. The user who likes to keep an eye on everything can set up the memory gauge, a clock, alarm systems and a series of other functions. In this way, all the best bits of the *Windows* system are readily to hand. *Dashboard* is stylish and neat as well as being an efficient way of keeping everything under control and working with *Windows* in the fastest possible way.

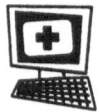

Help

What do the *Windows* files do?

When *Windows* is installed, there are huge numbers of files in the *Windows* directory. Here is a list of what the main ones do. You need this information if you are short of disk space and plan to delete files. Do **not** delete these.

HIMEM.SYS	Allocates extended memory
WIN.COM	Loads *Windows* DOS extender
DOSX.EXE	DOS extender for standard mode
WIN386.EXE	DOS extender for enhanced mode
KRNL286.EXE	Standard mode kernel
KRNL386.EXE	Enhanced mode kernel
GDI.EXE	Controls graphics device interface
USER.EXE	Controls user interface
*.DRV	Standard mode device drivers
*.386	Enhanced mode device drivers
SYSTEM.INI	Specifies system setup
WINOLDAP.MOD	Runs DOS apps in
~WOA*.*	Standard mode swap file
WIN386.SWP	Enhanced mode temporary swap file
	Enhanced mode permanent swap file
386SPART.PAR	Pointer to 386SPART.PAR
SPART.PAR	A hidden file linked to the swap file

Tip

If you are short of hard disk space, you may want to delete some *Windows* files.

To save some space, the following files can be deleted safely. If you are only ever going to run *Windows* in standard mode (and this is fairly unlikely, so proceed with caution) you can delete the following files:

CGA40WOA.FON
SGA80WOA.FON
SPWIN386.CPL
DOSAPP.FON
EGA40WOA.FON
EGA80WOA.FON

KRNL386.EXE
*.3GR
*.386
WIN386.EXE
WIN386.PS2
WINOA386.MOD

If you are only ever going to work in enhanced mode, you can delete the following:

DOSX.EXE
DSWAP.EXE
KRNL286.EXE
*.2GR
WINOLDAP.MOD
WSWAP.EXE

Tip

Don't forget basic DOS commands if you move to *Windows*.

Windows is graphically oriented and this means that you quickly become dependent on using the mouse and pull-down menus. Remember, though, that (for the moment, at least), *Windows* runs inside DOS. That means that DOS is always 'sitting behind' *Windows* and *Windows* programs. Bear in mind that, at some point, you may need or want to use basic DOS commands, such as *mem* or *copy*. You may also want to use the DOS editor *Edit* to make changes to your CONFIG.SYS and AUTOEXEC.BAT files. Try to keep in touch with DOS and *Windows*.

Tip

What to do if *Widows* won't run.

Not being able to start *Windows* at all can be very frustrating and there are a number of reasons why this may happen. Venditto (1992) offers the following suggestions as to why this may happen and what to do about the situation:

1. DOS may not be able to find file WIN.COM. Try switching to the directory where *Windows* is stored and typing WIN at the DOS

prompt. If this solves the problem, edit your AUTOEXEC.BAT file to include the *Windows* directory in the path statement. For example, if WIN.COM is in the directory C:\WINDOWS, your path statement should read PATH=C:\WINDOWS (make sure each directory in your path statement is separated by a semicolon).

2. There may not be enough available memory. Remove memory-resident programs by rebooting your system (press CTRL-ALT-DEL). If the problem persists, check the amount of available memory; in versions of DOS through 3.3 you can do this by running CHKDSK, which is usually stored in the DOS directory. (If it's not there, it will be on one of the DOS disks.) In versions of DOS starting with 4.0, you can also type MEM at any DOS prompt. Either DOS command tells you how much RAM is available. If you have less than 350K of available memory, you should edit your AUTOEXEC.BAT file to remove memory-resident programs that load automatically. You can run these programs after *Windows* is loaded, as you need them and according to the amount of available memory.

3. You may have changed hardware. Since *Windows* must have the correct device drivers installed for the video adapter in the system, it will not run if the wrong video display driver is installed. Run Setup by typing SETUP at the DOS prompt from the main *Windows* directory and change the hardware settings.

4. One of the *Windows* configuration files may have become corrupted. Run Setup from the main *Windows* directory and reinstall *Windows* in the directory where it was previously installed.

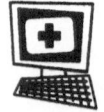

Help

Buying *Windows* software

Stephens (1993) offers the following set of tips for 'pain-free *Windows* software purchasing':

1. Define your requirements – do you really need all those features?
2. Make sure that your potential purchase plays by the *Windows* rules and conventions.
3. Look out for innovative ideas, but beware of overcomplicated user interfaces.
4. Make sure that any new software is compatible with your old.

5. Try out a demonstration version if you can.
6. Don't buy the first version of any program – wait a few weeks for the bug fixes.
7. Read the computer press (and bulletin boards if you have a modem) for other users' opinions of any potential purchase.
8. If you're not an experienced user, check out a product's technical support.
9. Shop around: never pay the recommended retail price.
10. Keep an eye out for competitive upgrades.

There is a variety of shareware programs available for *Windows*.

Tip

As we have noted elsewhere in this book, shareware offers you the chance to 'try before you buy'. Here are some of the *Windows* shareware programs that are available and which may be of use to a variety of health care users.

Above and Beyond

This is a remarkably sophisticated PIM – personal information manager – that is ideal for storing all the things that would otherwise go in your diary. You can store things to do, phone calls to make, lists of names and addresses and so on. If you have a modem, you can also have Above and Beyond dial the phone for you.

The program is simple to operate but allows you to set up a range of alarms and reminders. All types of recurring activities need be entered just once. You can print schedules to take your plans wherever you go. Includes a pop-up calendar, alarms, task and event timers, week and month at a glance, contact database and much more.

Like all shareware, there is a fee to pay to the author of the program if you continue to use it after the evaluation period.

WinBatch

This is a batch program maker that can help you to automate a range of *Windows* tasks. It is a sophisticated program that allows you to create sophisticated 'macros' or shortcuts to bring together a range of operations. You need to know a little about *Windows* to use this program but if you are used to DOS macro and shortcut developers, WinBatch will present you with few difficulties. Version 4.0 adds over 75 new functions, bringing the total to around 300. Many brand new functions for *Windows* 3.1 including DDE, network, multimedia, file attribute, system info, INI maintenance and much more.

Tommy Software CAD Draw 1.11a

This a major shareware release from Tommy Software in Berlin, the authors of Megapaint for DOS. If you need to do complicated drawings on the computer, this is a program to consider.

TS CAD Draw is a top class fully featured and powerful object oriented CAD/drawing package for *Windows* 3.1. It features a stunning range of drawing functions (including ellipse, ellipse arc, ellipse ring, parabola, zigzag line, circle arc chain, Bézier chain, spline and outline) and powerful manipulation functions including copy, move, scale, rotate, reflect, sheer and centre. The program supports up to 256 drawing layers, each of which can be individually faded out, frozen or displayed in a certain colour. It is possible to define a pen for each layer, which defines the line width, line colour and line pattern of all objects that will be drawn in this layer. All input is done with the mouse or the keyboard via a context-sensitive direct input, i.e. at any time a dialogue box can be opened which refers to the current command and enables you to input data.

A wide range of units of length and angle are supported. Built-in construction functions like perpendicular on circle, parallel variable, and parallel fixed, construction tangents, etc. are included multiple copy, rotation, distance, circle, array, freely configurable hatch functions, different types of grid settings, up to 900 symbols in a library – the feature list is considerable.

Winzip 5

This is a 'front end' for the popular file compression programs PKZIP and/or ARJ, LHARC.3.1 ASP. These programs are useful for compressing individual or batches of files so that they take up much less room on your hard disk. Alternatively, you may use the programs to squeeze more onto floppy disks. Many manufacturers use them to put programs onto fewer disks.

In the past, you were required to type fairly complicated commands at the DOS prompt in order to compress files using these programs. Winzip 5 offers a simple *Windows* interface for them. It is intuitive and easy to use and will be popular with anyone who needs to free space on their hard disks but who is not prepared to use a hard disk compression program.

All of the above programs are available from Omicron Systems Ltd, 45 Blenheim Crescent, Leigh on Sea, Essex SS9 3DT, telephone 0702-710391, who also supply a comprehensive on-disk catalogue of shareware programs.

Tip

Set up a permanent swap file.

A swap file allows *Windows* to work in 'virtual memory' mode. Put simply, when *Windows* runs out of memory, it checks with your hard disk to see if there is a swap file. If there is, that swap file is used as an extension to the computer's memory. Data can be temporarily shipped out to the swap file and then called back into memory as needed. There are two types of swap files: temporary and permanent. The permanent variety works faster.

To set up a permanent swap file, double click on the 386 enhanced icon in the control panel. In the 386 enhanced dialogue box, click on the virtual memory button and set the swap file to 'permanent'. Also, click the box that says 'Use 32-Bit Disk Access'. In most cases, this makes the use of the swap file more efficient. In just a very few cases, use of this feature makes the computer crash. If this happens, simply go back to this point and 'click off' the 'Use 32-Bit Disk Access' box.

Tip

Use a plain colour as a background instead of wallpaper.

Wallpaper – what you see 'behind' all the *Windows* boxes – eats into the computer's memory. As a rule, it is best to deselect any wallpaper that is in use. This is done via the control panel's 'Desktop' feature. Most of the time, of course, you don't see the wallpaper anyway.

Tip

Use lower resolution graphics.

Although high resolution graphics – Super VGA (800×600 pixels) – can make what is on the screen look clearer, it also means that what you see on the screen is smaller. Also, Super VGA runs more slowly. You may find an improvement on speed and readability if you stick to a standard VGA video setting – 640×480 pixels.

Tip

Disable expanded memory unless you really need it.

Windows does not use expanded memory. If you use a mixture of DOS and *Windows* programs you may need you computer configured to have both extended and expanded memory. If you only use *Windows* programs, disable any expanded memory. This can be done with third-party memory managers or with DOS's own *Memmaker* program.

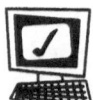

Tip

Shut down programs that you are not using.

It is tempting to open up a variety of programs under *Windows* and then to leave them running 'in the background'. This uses up the computer's memory. To run things faster, close down the programs that you are not using.

Tip

Windows contains its own wordprocessor that is useful if you are short of space.

If you are short of memory or hard disk space, you may want to consider using the *Write* wordprocessor that comes with *Windows*. Although it is not as fully featured as many of the other commercial wordprocessing packages, if all you need is a simple means of entering text, *Write* can be very useful. It is particularly useful if you require a compact text editing program when on the move. *Write* can be used with a notebook computer to provide a simple and effective way of producing text. It is handy, for example, if you use a larger wordpro-cessor on your desktop computer and have *Windows* on your notebook but limited hard disk space. The text files that *Write* produces are very versatile and can quickly be inserted into your desktop wordprocessing program.

Tip

Windows contains a simple but useful database program.

There is nothing particularly sophisticated about *Cardfile* which comes as part of the *Windows* set of programs. On the other hand, it is surprisingly useful and easy to use as a replacement for a 'real' cardfile. If you have a set of cards on your desk for references or names and addresses, consider using *Cardfile*. It is much easier to use than many other database programs and will be all that is needed by many people.

Tip

Work with maximized windows.

Although it can sometimes seem an attractive option to see various programs running at the same time by making each program's windows smaller, this also makes *Windows* run more slowly. As far as possible, work with each program filling all of the available screen. Use the ALT-TAB switch to move between open programs.

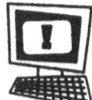

Trap

Windows often runs faster in standard mode.

Most people who have the appropriate computer and the required amount of memory run *Windows* in enhanced mode. However, if you are running a single program on a regular basis, you may find that standard mode is much quicker – it certainly loads more quickly. To start *Windows* in standard mode, type win/s at the DOS prompt. If you work with a 286 computer, you will have to use standard mode.

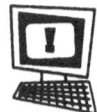

Trap

Don't forget *Character Map*.

Hidden away in the Accessories group window is a small application called *Character Map*. You can use this to see which characters are available with a particular font (or typeface) family. If you fire up *Character Map*, all of the characters are displayed on the screen in a box.

You can also select individual characters from *Character Map* while working in other programs.

Tip

Install more memory.

If you are short of birthday present ideas, ask for memory for your computer (RAM). *Windows* can use all the memory you can buy. The minimum usually recommended for running *Windows* successfully is 4Mb but it runs even better with 8Mb. RAM is easy to install, it usually just requires pushing into a range of slots inside your computer's box. Even if you can are not an electrical do-it-yourself fanatic, you can install extra memory.

Tip

Use a disk cache.

A disk cache speeds up reading from and writing to your hard disk. *Windows* comes with an excellent cache called *Smartdrive*. This is installed by inserting the following line in your AUTOEXEC.BAT file: C:\Windows\Smartdrv.exe. Note the spelling of this line. It is easy to type Smartdrive.exe and then to wonder why an error message appears on the screen every time you restart your computer!

Tip

Use the most up-to-date versions of *SmartDrive* and COMMAND.COM.

These two files are often updated with new versions of *Windows*. Make sure that you are using the most recent versions for best performance.

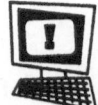

Trap

Use *Windows* versions of these files, not DOS versions.

Both of the above files are supplied with both DOS and *Windows*. If in doubt, when running *Windows* always use the *Windows* versions of the files. If you try to use the wrong version, you will usually get an error message on the screen telling you that that is what you have done.

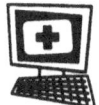

Help

Should you switch to *Windows for Workgroups*?

Windows for Workgroups is a version of *Windows* that is largely for those using networked computers. However, there are numerous benefits for the 'single user' who is not attached to a network. Gann (1993) suggests the following reasons for upgrading to *Windows for Workgroups*:

1. Disk performance. The new 32-bit File Access device driver makes your hard disk really fly, improving performance by about 50%.
2. Fax support. If you have a fax modem you can share it and fax from within your workgroup.
3. Remote access. Handy if you're at a remote site and need to download a data file.
4. Improved network drivers. The new range of network drivers make it a lot easier to connect to other networks, especially Novell Net Ware.
5. Improved File and Print Manager. *Windows* 3.1 users will like the new tool bars.
6. Wider video support. *Windows* now has a wide range of generic video drivers for Super VGA resolutions, such as 800×600 and 1024×768.
7. Better security. A user's configuration file is now encrypted and can't easily be bypassed.
8. Better admin. It's now possible to configure *Windows for Workgroups* 3.11 centrally.
9. Wider network support. You can hook up to a wider range of networking systems – connectivity to Net Ware is much better.
10. Better messaging and chat. You can now get messages from the Print Manager telling you your print is done.

Help

Should you switch to *Windows NT*?

Windows NT (new technology) is a specialist operating system produced by Microsoft and features full 32-bit technology. It is not, however, for the everyday user. Stephens (1994) offers the following checklist:

Should I be Using *Windows NT*?

YES	NO
I need to develop 32-bit programs.	I write programs in Visual Basic.
I need to create large database solutions.	I use standard productivity applications.
I want to control my corporate network.	I run a standard PC with 8Mb or less of RAM.
I use vertical-market programs which are available for *Windows NT*.	I need access to Adobe Type Manager fonts.
I need powerful security features.	I want to use a shell other than Program Manager.
I want to run huge hard disks or RAID subsytems.	I need stable drivers for my graphics accelerator.

If you are using an ordinary computer for ordinary programs like a wordprocessor and basic spreadsheet or database program, the answer to the question 'Should I change to *Windows NT*?' is probably 'no'.

Tip

Change the default directory of your favourite programs.

Often, *Windows* programs – particuarly wordprocessors – default to a particular directory. This means that the directory that is 'current' and to which you can save files is a **particular** one, decided by the software manufacturers. You can change this default directory very easily within the Program Manager. First, make sure the icon for the program is highlighted within the Program Manager. Next, from the File menu, open up the selection called 'Properties'. Then, in the section called 'Working Directory', type in the directory that you want to use as the default. You may, for example, keep all your wordprocessing data files in a directory called 'Papers'. If this was the case and you wanted your wordprocessor to automatically save files to this directory, you would type in c:\papers in the 'Working Directory' section.

You can have different working directories for different programs. This can be a useful way of organizing your files. You may, for example, set your database program to default to a directory called 'Data' and your graphics program to default to 'Graphics'. In this way, all the files associated with a particular type of program are saved, automatically, to a particular directory and not necessarily to the one determined by the manufacturers of the software.

This tip is not often documented in the literature and the manuals but it can make a considerable difference to the way in which you work with *Windows* programs.

Tip

Use *WinClock* to show the date and time.

WinClock is an excellent shareware program that allows you to display the date and time in the title bar of your *Windows* programs – including the Program Manager of *Windows*. The information displayed can also include the amount of space left on your hard disk and the amount of available memory. You can customize the display to show the information at the right or left ends of the title bar or you can 'toggle' the information on and off. In this case, a click of the mouse displays the information and another click hides it again. Although *Windows* offers you various clock functions, this is perhaps the neatest way of always displaying the time and date. If you want the program to start up each time you switch on your computer, you simply place a copy of the program's icon in the *Windows* Start-up directory.

Tip

Click on *Windows* title bars to decrease the size of the open window.

This is a useful shortcut. With *Windows* Program Manager and with most other *Windows* programs, you can 'shrink' the current open window a little by double clicking the left hand mouse button on the title bar of the window. Double clicking a second time resizes the window to fill the screen. This method is useful if you want to see what other windows are open 'underneath' the current one.

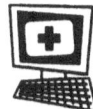

Help

Customize various features in *Windows* with the Control Panel.

One of the icons in the main window of *Windows* is called Control Panel. This allows you to make numerous changes to various aspects of

Table 5.2

Icon	Function
Color (*Windows* uses the American spelling)	Customize the *Windows* screen colours
Fonts	Load and unload different fonts or typefaces
Ports	Configure the serial ports COM1 to COM4
Mouse	Make changes to the way in which the mouse works
Desktop	Add and remove wallpaper, install a screensaver and modify the icons that you use
Keyboard	Set the keyboard to work with a particular language and change the keyboard's responsiveness
Printers	Install or remove various printer drivers
International	Select international formats for date, time and currency
Date/time	Set the time and day displayed by your computer
386 enhanced	Customize the settings for a computer containing a 386 or 486 processor chip. Change the settings for the swapdisk
Drivers	Add or remove drivers for sound cards and video players
Sound	Assign sound to different *Windows* events
MidiMapper	Configure sound boards for multimedia functions
Networks	Perform network specific changes

the *Windows* environment and it pays to become familiar with the various icons that are displayed when you double click on the Control Panel icon. The functions are identified in Table 5.2.

Tip

Start *Windows* as soon as you turn on your computer.

In order to allow *Windows* to start every time you switch your computer on, you need to add a line to your AUTOEXEC.BAT file. You do this with a text editor. Before you add the line, make sure that you have a backup of your AUTOEXEC.BAT file. This is essential to the proper running of your computer so only make this change if you know how to use a text editor. Normally, you cannot easily make this change using your wordprocessor.

The line that you add to your AUTOEXEC.BAT file is a simple one that reads as follows: Win. It must be the last line in your AUTOEXEC.BAT file and there should be no punctuation marks before or after the line.

Tip

Leave *Windows* and *Windows* programs quickly.

You do not have to call up the file menu and then click on the Close Menu item to leave *Windows* or *Windows* programs. Simply double click the mouse on the 'handle' at the left hand end of the title bar. This will bring up a submenu which checks that you really want to leave *Windows* or the *Windows* program. Confirm by clicking OK or by pressing the return (Enter) key.

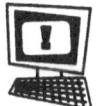

Trap

Don't run DOS utility programs through *Windows*.

If you need to use programs that check the integrity of your hard disk or which defragment your hard disk, do not use these by using the icon which takes you temporarily to DOS. Instead, exit *Windows* completely before you run these sorts of programs. One of the few exceptions to this is the program *PC-Tools for Windows* which contains a hard disk defragmentation program which can be run within *Windows*.

Tip

If you need to change your AUTOEXEC.BAT and/or CONFIG.SYS files regularly, there is a built-in *Windows* text editor.

Although it is not documented in the manual, *Windows* contains a text editor for editing AUTOEXEC.BAT, CONFIG.SYS and various other *Windows* control files. Only use it if you are sure that you know what you are doing! To install *Sysedit* into the main window of the Program Manager, follow these steps:

1. from the Edit menu, select New;
2. from the New menu, select Program Item;
3. fill in the following details on the menu that appears:

Description	Sysedit
Command Line	Sysedit.exe
Working Directory	c:\windows
Shortcut Key	None

These will ensure that a new icon is created which will give you access to *Sysedit*. *Sysedit* allows you to modify the following files:

- AUTOEXEC.BAT
- CONFIG.SYS
- win.ini
- system.ini.

You must make backups of the four systems files before you change them.

Trap

The files that are accessed by *Sysedit* (see previous tip) are essential to the running of your computer and to the proper running of *Windows* and you **must** have backup copies of them before you change them in any way. Make sure that these backups are on a floppy disk and then, if you make any mistakes in editing the files, you can be sure that you can always 'rescue' your setup.

RECOMMENDED READING

Gookin, D. (1993) *Microsoft Guide to Optimising Windows*, Microsoft Press. Available from Computer Manuals, 50 James Road, Tyseley, Birmingham B11 2BA. Telephone: 021-706-1188

This is a very readable and extremely useful guide to just about every aspect of managing *Windows*. It starts with an authoritative and very well written chapter on configuring DOS for *Windows* and there is much here that you won't find in the manuals. The next chapter explains the more arcane details of the *Windows* start-up files. Again, this sort of information is not readily available in the literature that accompanies *Windows* and it is good to have it so clearly explained. Following chapters deal with optimizing *Windows* and, for once, there is clear advice about whether or not to have a RAM file and how to set up your CONFIG.SYS and AUTOEXEC.BAT files to make sure that *Windows* runs most efficiently. Later chapters deal with DOS programs running under *Windows*, multitasking configurations, networks, tele-communication and faxes.

It is possible that you could learn the information contained in this book by reading the computer journals and spending your evenings working through the thick manuals. What Gookin has achieved is an entertaining – yes, the book is amusing as well as readable – guide to everything to do with *Windows* and all in a reasonably priced volume. This is not one of the 'doorstop' computer books but a concise and extremely useful handbook.

6 Tips and traps in managing files

You must organize your files, especially if you are using a hard disk and, these days, most people do. This chapter offers tips and traps in organizing files on your hard disk. At the risk of being repetitive, the point that must be made over and over again is that you must backup your files.

Be methodical in planning your hard disk organization.

These days, almost all computers have hard disks and an increasing number of them have large hard disks. It is vitally important that you do not simply empty all of your files into the root directory of your disk. The root directory is the first and main directory of the hard disk – it is usually called the C: drive. You must have subdirectories branching off the hard disk. All computer programs contain many files. You are likely to have a variety of programs on your hard disk at any given time along with a variety of data files that you produce with those programs. If you have all of those files in the root directory, you won't know which files work with which programs. That means that if you want to remove a program from your hard disk, you won't know which files to remove.

Nowadays, almost all programs install themselves directly into subdirectories that are set up by the installation element of the program. For example, if you install *Word for Windows*, the installation routine opens up a subdirectory called *C:\Winword* into which the main program files are installed. *Word for Windows* also sets up other sub-directories within C:\Winword to contain other files.

The planning that you have to do is how to organize your data files

– the files that you produce with your wordprocessor, spreadsheet or graphics program. It is useful to set up a variety of subdirectories that suit the data that you produce. You might, for example, use a range of subdirectories as follows.

C:\letters (letters)
C:\records (patient, client or student records)
C:\work (work related files)
C:\home (home related files).

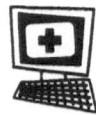

Help

Understanding directories.

The terms 'directories' and 'subdirectories' are often used synonymously. Essentially, the system works like this. You start with the main 'directory' of your hard disk (known as the root directory and usually referred to as the C: drive). This can be compared to a filing cabinet.

Within this root directory, you can organize 'diectories' or 'subdirectories' such as the ones referred to in the previous tip (C:\work and C:\letters). These can be compared to the drawers in the filing cabinet – they allow you to keep various documents (or files) together in one place. Beneath these directories, you can develop further subdirectories. Within the directory C:\letters, for example, you could have a number of subdirectories such as 'band', 'health' and 'personal'. The 'addresses' of these subdirectories would be as follows.

C:\letters\bank
C:\letters\health
C:\letters\personal.

These subdirectories can be compared to the various cradles that can be placed in filing cabinet drawers to further organize your files. In theory – and even in practice – you can continue to develop further levels of subdirectories. You could, for example, have another set of subdirectories in the 'health' directory but this is not recommended. Having lots of levels of subdirectories can be confusing and hard to negotiate your way around on the hard disk. You are advised to stick to one or two levels of subdirectories. I find that I can cope quite easily with the following range of directories for containing my data files:

- C:\Phil (this contains any personal files, including my CV, personal letters, tax documents and so forth);
- C:\Masters (this contains files relating to the range of Masters degrees that I organize in my work at the university);
- C:\Phd (this contains files relating to the doctoral program that I am responsible for);
- C:\Handouts (this contains handouts and slides for use when teaching);
- C:\Overseas (this contains files to do with a range of courses that I run in other countries);
- C:\Articles (this contains manuscripts for papers and articles submitted to journals);
- C:\Books (this contains book manuscripts). I also have subdirectories within C:\Books containing each manuscript. For example, the subdirectory for this book is C:\Book\compute2. The subdirectory C:\Book\compute1 contains all the chapters for my other computing book *Personal Computing for Health Professionals*.

All the other directories and subdirectories on my hard disks contain program files. I have yet to find any reason to open more directories for containing data files.

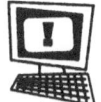

Trap

You must backup your work!

This is the most important thing in the book. You must backup all new files that you create. Hard disks do not last for ever and at some time, yours will fail. Sometimes, too, it is possible to accidentally wipe files off your hard disk. I once accidentally erased a chapter of my PhD thesis. Over the years, I have also lost a range of smaller files. Why? Because I didn't have backup copies on floppy disk. Now, I always make backups and I use a tape streamer (see below). You simply cannot take chances. Make sure that any data files that are on your hard disk are also available on floppies or on some other backup medium.

You don't really have to backup your program files. You already have a set of a backup disks in the form of the original disks that were supplied by the software company. However, chances are you have customized those programs to quite a considerable degree. You may, for example, have added all sorts of words to the spell checker in your wordprocessor. You have two choices here. If you know the files that these changes are recorded in, you can just backup those files. If you don't know the names of the 'custom' files, the safest bet is to backup all your program files as well. This again is easier if you use a tape streamer.

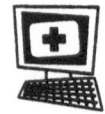

Help

Backing up your data: good practice.

It is important to be methodical and organized in working out your data backup strategy. Norfolk (1993) offers the following ten tips for good parctice:

1. Use data compression, fast utilities and automatic schedulers to make backups as painless as possible. This will help ensure the backup is done.
2. Exit programs or log everybody off the network (as appropriate) while backups run.
3. Backup media can fail too: keep a cycle of old backups and store backups in clean, dry, cool, dark conditions.
4. Validate backups: use error correction facilities and try regular test restores of random files.
5. Keep at least one backup generation where it isn't exposed to the same risks as the original data. This will usually mean storing off-site.
6. Unprotected backups are a classic way of breaking into a system to steal data or install rogue codes. Keep them locked up.
7. Clearly label and mark your backups so you can find your backup data when needed.
8. Make use of the write-protect tab on floppy disks to prevent accidental erasure of your backup data.
9. If you have a network, store data centrally on the file server and have procedures for backing up the server.
10. In a business, make someone specifically responsible for backup procedures and making sure that everything important is backed up.

Tip

For larger hard disks, use a tape streamer.

When hard disks averaged 20 or 40Mb, it was possible to backup data files to floppy disks. A high density floppy disk can hold a little over 1Mb of data. That means if half of your 40Mb hard disk is taken up with data files, you will need about 20 floppies to backup all of those files. With larger hard disks – and *Windows* programs often mean that you need a larger hard disk – you need another approach to backing up. Probably the cheapest and easiest option is to use a **tape streamer**. This is a device that either fits into your computer box or sits in its own box next to the computer and contains the means of backing up your data to a miniature tape cassette. The process is fairly fast – many tape streamers backup at a rate of more than 10Mb a minute and tapes are fairly hardwearing. The software that runs these machines is also simple to operate and you can make a daily backup of any new files at the end of every day or at the end of any given working session. You can ask the software to make an incremental backup and thus backup only those files that have been changed or new files that you have created.

The only apparent disadvantage with tape streamers is that they tend to be noisy – they sound very like a dentist's drill when they are operating. For this reason, you may not want to do large backups during working hours, but even this can be taken care of. Most tape streamers can be set so that they backup your files, automatically, at a preset time. Thus, you could set yours to backup all new and modified files at 2.00 am. In this way, the tape streamer does all the work while you are away (or asleep). If you are doubtful about the efficiency of this system, you can always check that the backup has been achieved in the morning. This approach means that you must leave the computer on all the time. You can, of course, turn off the monitor but the main box must be left on. As we have noted in an earlier chapter, many authorities suggest that it is better to leave the computer on all the time, anyway. It is the power surges that occur when you turn your computer on and off that cause wear and tear to components.

Tip

Maximize the efficiency of your tape streamer.

The fastest way of operating a tape streamer is to have it **streaming**. Streaming is said to occur when the data coming off the hard disk is being written to the tape at the same rate. A tape that is streaming will be driven continuously. A tape that is not streaming will constantly stop and start and thus take longer to complete the backup process. Streaming can usually be achieved by turning off all data compression facilities. This, of course, will mean that you can store less data on any given tape. There is always a choice between the amount of data that can be stored on a tape and the time that is taken to complete a backup. Streaming is very desirable when large amounts of data have to be backed up.

Tip

Most backup systems allow you to use a password.

One of the reasons for backing up data from a hard disk is to protect that data. If data is very sensitive – patient or client notes are an example – use a password to protect your computer and your backups.

Tip

Develop a 'fail-safe' backup policy.

There are various ways of organizing backup procedures. One system is to do a complete backup of all the files on the hard disk once a week and then to do incremental backups on every other day of the week. An incremental backup is one in which only new or changed files are backed up. Most backup programs and tape streamers can organize incremental backups.

Many would argue that it is important to do two full backups a week and to store one of them away from the health care centre. In this way, you have a complete set of the contents of your computer that can be restored to a new computer should anything happen to the one you are using. Bear in mind that you can only do incremental backups if you have first done a full backup at some point. Remember, too, that if you leave a lot of time between full backups, your incremental backups will become greater in number and this may make restoration of data more difficult. It is a good plan to do a total backup once a week at a particular time of day so that it becomes a routine. I make a habit of setting my work tape streamer to do a full backup every Friday lunchtime. Usually, by the time I have returned from lunch, the whole of the hard disk is backed up. I then do incremental backups every afternoon before I leave work (see the next tip). Another method, as we have seen, is to use a scheduling program to do automatic backups while you are away from the computer.

Tip

Keep one set of backups off-site.

Offices, hospitals, clinics and colleges get burgled. It is one thing to lose your computer – that can usually be replaced. No amount of backing up will work if you lose the backup media. If you keep all your tapes or all your backup disks next to your computer, if your place of work is burgled you stand to lose all your data.

It is a good policy to have one set of backup files or tapes off-site. I make it a practice to backup my hard disk at work, completely, once a week to a tape streamer. I make two copies of the backup; one I store at work, the other I take home. In this way, I always have one complete copy of what is on my hard disk away from work.

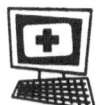

Help

Other forms of backup media.

Many people use floppy disks or tape streamers to backup their data but there are other media for use in the backup process. Here are two of the more common ones:

- Removable hard disks. Like floppy disks and tapes, these can be taken away from the computer and stored at another location. They rely on your having either a computer containing a special slot for removal disks or an external unit that houses one. Duplicate removal hard disks can be expensive.

- Optical storage. These are more expensive and use specially prepared disks for storage. They can be used to store very large amounts of data and may be an ideal choice for larger health care organizations that rely on a network.

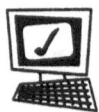

Organize groups of files by number.

Tip

If you are writing sections of a report or chapters of a book, make sure that you 'name' the files containing each section or chapter so that they appear, in order, in any file management program that you use. For example, I have stored the files for this book as follows:

000front.doc (the opening pages, including the title and contents pages)
00intro.doc (the Introduction)
01buy.doc (Chapter 1)
02soft.doc (Chapter 2)
03mach.doc (Chapter 3)
04dos.doc (Chapter 4)
05window.doc (Chapter 5)
06files.doc (Chapter 6)
07wrdpro.doc (Chapter 7)
08datab.doc (Chapter 8)
09write.doc (Chapter 9)
10resear.doc (Chapter 10)
11books.doc (Appendix)
12refs.doc (References)

There are a few points to note about this sort of naming. First, if the files are numbered in this style, they will appear in order in any file listing. Second, the short names in each file label tells me what is in each file. If, on the other hand, you simply name your files '1', '2', '3' and so forth, when you get to '10', that file will be listed before '1'. Also, this form of naming tells you nothing about what is in each file.

All of these files are contained in their own subdirectory called *1Compute*. The '1' at the front of this subdirectory name ensures that the subdirectory will also be listed first in any file manager listing of directories and subdirectories. This gives me quicker access to the book project while I am working on it. Once I have completed writing and editing the manuscript, all the files will be moved to a subdirectory called C:\books\compute. In this way, they will be filed away with other book manuscripts but still in their own subdirectory.

Organize your files and the rest of your work with a personal information manager.

A personal information manager (PIM) takes the place of your diary, address book, cardfile and any other methods that you have of organizing your personal work. *PackRat* (Polaris Software) is an example of such a manager. It will help you to organize your computer files and all the information referred to above.

PackRat looks complicated when you first open it up. It relies heavily on the use of objects and these are described in Chapter 5. Essentially, *PackRat* contains a large number of predefined objects which you can customize to suit the way that you work. There are, for examples, objects which will contain your phone book, 'to do' lists and contact lists. There are others to contain a list of your computer files and these are linked to the programs that run them. This means that you simply click on the file and that file is automatically opened up inside the program that runs it. Other objects produce Gannt charts, diaries, clocks and a variety of alarm systems.

All of these objects can be contained within various 'folders'. A folder, in this case, refers to a single screen. Each new folder (or new screen) is accessed by clicking on a tab at the top of the screen. Each folder can 'contain' a variety of objects that you choose from a menu. You might, for example, have a folder marked Phone Book, which contained a list of all your names and addresses, a quick-contact reminder list of people you need to call and a clock. Another folder, perhaps marked Programs, could contain icons that represent all your programs – *PackRat* allows you to link all your programs to itself in this way. Yet another folder could contain job-specific objects such as a diary and a 'to do' list.

Some PIMs simply act as on-screen diary replacements. *PackRat* is much more than this. It is a highly customizable information manager that can help any health professional to organize his or her work more effectively. The program opens to a variety of preset folders but do not be put off by their complicated appearance. Almost everything that you see on the opening screens can be customized to suit the way you work. *PackRat* is worth persevering with – especially if you need a single program with which to organize and control all the files on your computer and all the work on your desk. In the end *PackRat* can replace the Program Manager of *Windows* and allow you to use your computer in much more flexible ways.

Buy a 'utilities' program.

Tip

PC Tools has always been a market leader in the utilities section. *PC-Tools for Windows* (Central Point Software) puts the product way ahead. So what is a 'utilities package'? It is a series of programs that you don't necessarily need every day but when you do need them, you need to know that they are going to work. Typically, utilities programs help you to recover lost data, to 'unformat' disks and to find deleted files. *PC-Tools for Windows* does all of these things and many more besides. Its *Windows* presentation also makes it a very attractive program to work with.

Listing all of the things that are contained in *PC-Tools for Windows* is difficult, there are so many. First, it has a replacement 'desktop' for *Windows*. You can use this in place of the Program Manager and it has a number of enhanced facilities. You can, for example, make use of 'multiple desktops' – you can develop a series of opening screens, all of which are different and which are tailored exactly to the way you work on different projects. Within this part of the program there are facilities for developing new icons, for changing the colour scheme and even the font sizes on the screen. Altogether, a powerful and sophisticated set of tools. Personally, I have always found the simplicity of the basic *Windows* setup to be more than adequate and I found this aspect of *PC-Tools for Windows* a bit of overkill. Perhaps it grows on you.

There is also a file management package that replaces the *Windows* file manager. This really is useful. It allows you to view all of your files and in most formats. Thus you can take a quick look at a graphics file in much the same way as you might a wordprocessing text file. This is a considerable improvement on most file organizers and viewers which can rarely view the sheer range of file formats that is the case with this program. Built into the new file manager is the ability to compress files and decompress them. Whilst there is a variety of third-party programs designed to do this, it is good to see a file compression program built into a file manager. Generally, the *PC-Tools* file manager is an excellent replacement for the *Windows* one.

PC-Tools has offered a defragmenting program for a number of years. The new *Windows* version works from within *Windows*. In the past, if your hard disk had become cluttered with bits of files dotted all over it, the only way to defragment it was to exit *Windows* and do the job via DOS. The new version not only works within the *Windows* environment but it also allows you to set up the defragmentation process to occur at regular intervals throughout the working day. If, for example, you set it to defragment at 30 minute intervals, then your hard disk will be automatically defragmented when you have a break from computing. I found this was particularly useful breaks. You can return from lunch to find that your hard disk has been optimized.

The program also contains a variety of tools for undeleting files that have been accidentally deleted. In fact, you can set the *Sentry* program in the package to monitor all the files you delete and to save them against the time when you may need to recover them. You can set the program up to flush out these saved files at a time frequency that you choose. Also, there are numerous facilities for backing up files from hard disks and other storage media.

Another part of the package offers extensive protection against virus invasion, while another lets you set up your computer to do preset tasks at particular times. If, for example, you need to backup your hard disk every day to a tape streamer, you can set the program to make this happen automatically during the evening or the early morning. In this way, you save yourself considerable time by freeing 'working hours'.

System Consultant, another element of the program, provides a detailed analysis of the computer that you are working on and offers you hints about optimizing the running of it. It also tells you the overall speed of your processor and hard disk in comparison with other similar computers. Finally in this shortlist of some of the elements of the program, *ScriptTools* offers a sophisticated but easy-to-use macro system that can help to automate various aspects of your day-to-day computer work.

So what is missing? For some reason, Central Point have decided to leave out the caching program *PC-Cache* from this version of *PC-Tools*. Instead, they recommend the use of *Smartdrive*, the caching facility supplied with *Windows*.

Overall, this is a comprehensive and exhaustive set of tools that are all brought together under a very well-designed *Windows* interface. Everyone needs a utilities package at some time. If you use *Windows* and are planning to buy such a package, this is the one to go for. Without doubt it is the best on the market.

RECOMMENDED READING

Miller, A.R. (1993) *The ABCs of DOS 6*, Sybex. Available from Computer Manuals, 50 James Road, Tyseley, Birmingham B11 2BA. Telephone: 021-706-1188

If you are new to computers, this is the book for you. Like all Sybex books (and most are available from Computer Manuals) this one is comprehensive and extremely well designed. The book is a teach-yourself-DOS course. Starting with first principles, it deals with all the main aspects of working with the operating system. You are shown how to name files, format disks and do all the housekeeping tasks that anyone who uses a PC needs to do. My one reservation is the author's detailed discussion of the DOS shell. The shell is a reasonably user-friendly menu system which sits between DOS and your programs. However, given the shift to *Windows*, I imagine that not all that many people use the shell any more. Miller's lessons make it almost essential that you use it to understand other features of DOS.

This is an ideal starting point for working with computers. It would make an ideal present for a person who has just been given a PC and it would be useful in a large health care institution as a book to put on the desks of those who have computers but are too scared to use them. Miller writes clearly and his lessons all include 'hands on' illustrations.

7 Tips and traps in wordprocessing

More people use personal computers for wordprocessing than for any other function. Most people, too, only use a small number of features in their wordprocessors. In this chapter, we explore ways in which you can exploit some of the features of your wordprocessor and make best use of it.

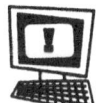

Trap

Wordprocessing is not typing.

Although your touch-typing skills, if you have them, will transfer to the computer, bear in mind that certain other conventions do not apply. The obvious difference is that you do not have to press 'Return' at the ends of lines – all wordprocessors offer you a 'word-wrap' feature which causes text to break at the ends of lines. Also, you should not type two spaces between sentences when using a wordprocessing program; it leads to an unnecessarily 'gappy' look to the text. If you were once a typist, however, this habit will be a very hard one to break. You may have to build yourself a 'clean up' macro which takes out all the second spaces. This sort of macro makes use of the Search and Replace feature of the wordprocessor and replaces every 'double space' that it finds with a 'single space'. The best sort of macro only replaces double spaces that it finds after a full stop, question mark or exclamation mark. In this way, intentional double spaces are retained.

Tip

Enter text first, arrange it later.

If you are using a *Windows* wordprocessor, you can save time by entering all your text – including headings, titles and other details – to the screen first. Once you have typed the whole of the document, you can return to concentrating on how the various elements of the text look. This method is much quicker than stopping to format as you type. Also, the chances are that this method will help you to be more consistent in your use of formatting features.

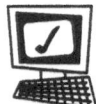

Tip

Simplicity is genius.

Use a simple layout for your text, whatever sort of document you are preparing. Many people are dazed by the amount of choice they have in changing the way documents look and end up with very messy documents. It is good desktop publishing and wordprocessing policy to keep everything simple. It also makes your final document much easier to read.

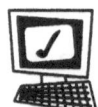

Tip

Stick to two fonts.

This is a corollary of the above tip. Don't get carried away by a choice of fonts (or typefaces). As a rule, use only two in any given document. It is usual to use one serif font and one sans serif for headings.

Tip

Consider using 'left justification' only.

It is tempting to go for the symmetrical look and to justify both the right and left margins. This may at first seem an attractive option but generally it is better practice only to justify the left margin. It is standard practice that correspondence makes use only of left justified text. Also, it is thought that left justified text is easier to read. The other term used for 'justified left' margin is 'ragged right'. The following two paragraphs demonstrate 'full justification' (right and left margins justified) and 'left justification'.

This is an example of a piece of text which is fully justified. With full justification, both margins are straight. This is fine if your wordprocessor can adjust the text appropriately but many run rivers of white space through your document if you justify both margins. Also, full justification is quite hard on the eye. It makes for too much symmetry and makes the text look like solid blocks.

This is an example of a piece of text which is left justified only. At first, it may seem the crude option – after all, it is not so neat as full justification. If, on the other hand, you have to proof read fully justified text it soon becomes apparent why many people feel it best only to use left justification. Try both. You can soon turn off the form of justification that you do not like.

Tip

Get your paragraphs right.

There are two standard ways of representing paragraphs in a document and these are illustrated below:

Style one

This is one method of producing paragraphs. With this approach, you simply leave two spaces between each paragraph. This is sometimes know as the 'block' method of paragraphing.

This is the second paragraph using this method. You will note that the new paragraph starts flush to the left hand margin. This is another feature of the 'block' style of paragraphing. It is popular in some types of report and it is sometimes used in business letters.

Style two

This is another method of producing paragraphs. With this approach, you begin the first paragraph flush to the left hand margin. No gap is left between paragraphs.

The second and subsequent paragraphs beneath any headings are indented and you will notice that this book is set with paragraphs of this sort.

This is another paragraph and you will notice that it, too, is indented from the left hand edge. This style is often used in books and journals and, increasingly, it is becoming a standard way of laying out work with the computer.

There is one style that sometimes arises when computer users are not clear about how to lay out paragraphs with a wordprocessor. It is to be avoided because it leads to 'blocks' of text in which it is difficult to recognize paragraph breaks at all. It is illustrated below.

Style three: the one to avoid

When people are new to wordprocessing, they often realize that they are liberated from pressing the 'Return' key at the ends of lines. They read in the manuals that the only time you need to press the 'Return' key is if you are starting a new paragraph. With this in mind, they start a new paragraph by only pressing the return key.

This leads to this sort of error. Here, the paragraph starts flush to the left hand margin but no extra lines are left between paragraphs and the first line of the new paragraph is not indented.

This is another new paragraph. As you can see, this approach leads to a block of text that is divided into paragraphs but, at first glance, it appears not to be so divided.

This is a common error of layout but it is one to be avoided if at all possible. Either use the 'block' style of paragraphing or the 'indent' style but do not mix the two.

Tip

Keep your documents short.

It is best to keep wordprocessing documents short. Large documents take longer to scroll through and make more demands on your computer's memory. If you are writing a long report or a thesis or book manuscript, divide it up into sections or chapters. Have each section or chapter as a separate file. Most of the larger wordprocessors make provision for all the chapters to be linked together before you print out. *WordPerfect for Windows* and *WordPerfect for DOS* are particularly good in this respect.

Tip

Write quickly, edit at leisure.

This is the point of wordprocessing that you can work quickly. Forget trying to make the first draft your last. Forget, too, correct spelling and layout. Feel free to type quickly and even to write in note form if this is what you prefer. You can return to your text later to edit – once the purple patch has passed.

Tip

Backup to the hard disk regularly.

Many wordprocessing programs have an automatic backup feature. But this is not always what it seems to be and is never a replacement for making regular backups to the hard disk. The automatic backup in *WordPerfect*, for example, means that your current document is always saved if there is a sudden power cut (the Americans refer to this as 'power outage!'). If this happens or if your computer 'hangs', then your document is safe. However, if you just exit the program in the normal way this backup file is lost. With this in mind, save your work to disk at frequent intervals. A good time to do this is 'between thoughts'. As you pause to think things through, hit the 'save' button or make yourself a macro and a button that can be clicked which automatically saves what is on the screen and returns you to the document. This must become a habit.

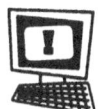

Trap

Make backups of all your data files.

This is the first and only law of wordprocessing. You **must** make backups of your data files. All the data that is on your hard disk must be backed up to floppies or to a tape. There are no exceptions to this rule. One day, your hard disk will fail or you will find that part of it has been corrupted. If that happens and you have not done regular backups, your data will be lost – forever! I speak from experience. I have, on two occasions, lost whole book chapters through not observing this rule. After the second loss, I bought a tape streamer and the last thing I do after a wordprocessing session is to backup new and modified files to tape.

Tip

Use the grammar checker and read style manuals.

Most of the bigger wordprocessors include a grammar checker as part of the package. Use these frequently – they are a useful way of trapping some of your grosser grammatical errors. You can learn a lot from a grammar checker. If you feel that yours is too pedantic, customize it. Most grammar checkers can themselves be edited to suit your style of writing.

Tip

Customize your wordprocessor to suit the way you work.

It is often said that most people only use 20% of their wordprocessing features 80% of the time. I am not sure that this is based on formal research but it does seem to be the case. The whole point of having a fully featured wordprocessor is to be able to use nearly all of the features. Find out what is included in yours.

Tip

Learn how to use macros.

Macros are shortcuts to commands. You can link a whole string of commands to one set of keystrokes or one button. An example of a macro would be one that calls up your letter layout. Another would turn on a particular format layout. Simple macros are also simple to develop. Learning how to make macros does not take very long and is worth the investment of time. On the other hand, do not be tempted to make huge numbers of macros. In the end, your time saving devices are likely to go unused if you make too many.

Tip

Learn how to use styles and style sheets.

Most wordprocessors offer you styles or style sheets. These are standard formats for paragraphs, sections of documents or even whole documents that can be applied at any time. Imagine, for example, that you have developed a standard way of laying out headings and titles of documents. If you save these as styles you will be able to use them again and again. Styles can save you a lot of time but, as with the macros, only make styles that you are going to use.

Tip

Use the *Windows* Print Manager.

As a rule, use the *Windows* Print Manager to route all your documents to the printer. If you do this, you free your wordprocessor more quickly because *Windows* takes over responsibility for printing out your document from your wordprocessor. Also, if you use the *Windows* Print Manager for all your *Windows* programs, you will find that you produce standardized work. With the *Windows* Print Manager, all the fonts that you have on your computer can be made available to all your *Windows* programs.

Tip

Work in single spacing.

This is an obvious tip but one that is often overlooked. Although you will want to print out certain sorts of documents double spaced (essays, article manuscripts, etc.), type them single spaced and do the double spacing later. This means that you will be able to see more text on the screen at any given time. It also means that your document can be scrolled through more quickly.

Tip

Use the file summary screen to record details of the contents of your files.

The file summary feature is a useful one that comes with many wordprocessors. It allows you to enter details about who typed a particular document, when it was opened for the first time, when it was last edited and a summary of what the document is about. With *Word for Windows* you can determine what form your file summary screen takes – the summary screen is fully customizable. You usually have to make an adjustment to the 'preferences' section of your wordprocessor to enable it to prompt you to fill in a file summary document every time you close a new file.

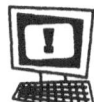

Trap

Indexing facilities in wordprocessors are limited.

Bear in mind that the index facility can only index documents that are produced and printed out from your wordprocessor. It cannot be used for proofs of manuscripts sent to you by editors or publishers. Also, indexing must be the very last thing you do to a document. If you index and then make changes to the document, your page numbering may not be correctly indexed.

Take frequent breaks.

Wordprocessors, like computers themselves, are sometimes too easy to use. When you are working well, it is tempting to sit and type for long periods. It is thought that one of the causes of repetitive strain injury is the sustained nature of the repetition. With typewriters, you had to stop every few minutes to put paper in the machine. With a wordprocessor, all you have to do is type. This can be a strain on the hands and wrists and it can also lead to bad posture and eye problems. Every five or ten minutes, stop typing and stretch. At least every hour, take a break away from the computer. Also, this is a more sociable way of working if you have to use a computer at home.

TIPS AND TRAPS FOR *WORDPERFECT FOR WINDOWS* (WORDPERFECT UK)

WordPerfect for Windows is an extremely comprehensive program that includes all the usual wordprocessing functions plus many more. It has developed considerably since its first edition and now boasts a spreadsheet function that can produce graphs and charts, an extensive array of preset document templates (known as *Express Docs*). *WordPerfect for Windows* will appeal to those who have used the best-selling DOS version of the program. It is hard to imagine how much further a wordprocessor can develop.

WordPerfect for Windows is currently available in version 6.0. Apart from all the usual wordprocessing functions, it offers extensive charting and drawing facilities. Now, pie charts, bar charts and a wide range of drawings can be developed and then inserted straight into your document. With a click of the mouse button you can produce boxes, columns and all the other features that are more often associated with desktop publishing programs. The keynote, though, is usability. One of the things that marks out this program is its ease of use. If you can use *Windows* you will soon be at home with *WordPerfect*. It is also almost infinitely customizable. One of its strongest features is its use of the button bar – a row of push buttons at the top of the screen that can be modified to suit the way you work. You can even add buttons that start up other programs. It seems highly likely that you could use *WordPerfect* as the program that is always on your screen. To move to other applications, you simply click a button. This not only makes for convenience but also for speed and efficiency of use.

WordPerfect for Windows 6.0 comes with a huge range of ready-to-use document templates known as *Express Docs*. This means that you can produce formal letters, fax sheets, memos and even a CV in few minutes and without having to plan the layout of such documents. Again, this will be an important feature for colleges and departments where standardization is important.

Are there any drawbacks? *WordPerfect for Windows 6.0* could occupy more than 30Mb of your hard disk if you install the whole program. Also, you need at least 4Mb of RAM in which to run it and 6Mb is recommended. Unfortunately, too, it is slow when compared to some other *Windows* products. On the other hand, it has yet to be beaten for its sheer range and number of easy-to-use features.

Tip

You can modify the button bar extensively.

Acerson (1992) identifies the following steps to explain how to add, delete or change the order of the buttons on the button bar:

- Choose View, Button Bar Setup and then Edit. The Edit Button Bar dialogue box appears. Notice that the mouse pointer changes to a hand holding a button.

- To delete a button, position the mouse pointer (the hand holding a button) on the button to be deleted and drag the button off the Button Bar. When you release the mouse, the button is deleted.

- To add a button, select the feature that is to be placed on a button – the same way you select it when working normally in *WordPerfect for Windows*. You can use the menus or the keyboard shortcuts. For example, to add a button that displays the *WordPerfect* Characters dialogue box, either select Font and then WP Characters or press CTRL+W.

- To move a button, position the mouse pointer on the button to be moved and drag it to a new location.

- To place the button between two other buttons, drag it so that it straddles the border between them.

- To place a button on either end of the button bar, drag it as far toward that end as it will go.
- Choose OK when you are satisfied with the arrangement of the button bar.
- When you add more buttons than will fit on one row, *WordPerfect* must scroll one or more of them off the screen. When that happens, left and right arrows appear to the left of the button bar. You can click on these arrows to scroll the button bar in either direction until you find the button you want.

Tip

You can add macros to the button bar.

The button bar feature also allows you to add a macro to a button. You may, for example, have developed a macro that calls up a particular document. This can be assigned its own button.

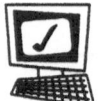

Tip

Consider showing only text on the button bar.

Button bar buttons are rather large in *WordPerfect for Windows*. You may want to use the 'text only' feature that shows only the name of the button rather than the name and a decorative icon.

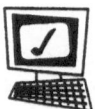

Tip

You can easily return to one of the four documents you last worked on.

If you click on the file menu at the top of the screen, you will find the names of the last four documents that you worked on listed at the bottom of that menu. By clicking on one of those names, you can recall it to the screen. This tip also works with *Word for Windows* and *AmiPro*.

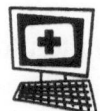

Help

You can buy add-on templates for *WordPerfect for Windows 5.2*.

Express Docs is an 'add-on' program for *WordPerfect for Windows 5.2* – version 6.0 includes these documents as part of the main program.

Express Docs integrates almost completely into that industry leading wordprocessor and offers the user an extra button bar. *WordPerfect* uses button bars to display frequently used operations and commands. With *Express Docs* installed, the user can choose from a wide range of beautifully produced and ready-made templates.

There are various templates for letters and memos, ranging from the formal to the informal. There are templates for fax sheets, invitations and slide presentations. There are still others for a wide range of reports and report covers. All you do is select the template you want, fill in the 'blanks' and you have a tailor-made and very professional looking document. No doubt you could produce similar results by yourself and without the aid of *Express Docs*. To do so, though, you would have to invest many hours of time in learning how to work with the more arcane desktop publishing features of *WordPerfect for Windows 5.2*. This is the quick way and easily the best way of working.

Also packaged with *Express Docs* are a series of document enhancement features. There are 'drop capitals', so that you can enlarge the first letter of your document. This is useful if you are producing newsletters or handouts. There is also a wide selection of different types of page borders. Again, such features are useful if you want to produce goodlooking documents with the minimum of fuss.

Express Docs is easily installed from a single disk. You need to be running *WordPerfect for Windows 5.2.* and then the rest is automatic. Definitely a product for health professionals who use *WordPerfect for Windows 5.2* on a regular basis.

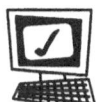

Tip

Manage large documents with the master document feature.

WordPerfect for Windows enables you to create a master document which calls up a series of other documents at the touch of a button. You can use this to draw together all the chapters of a book or all the sections of a report. Also, when you have finished working on the expanded document, you can save each section and its changes individually. *WordPerfect* offers what is probably the best way of managing larger projects.

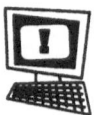

Trap

Macros in *WordPerfect for Windows* work differently to those in *WordPerfect for DOS*.

In *WordPerfect 5.1*, the macro facility worked by recording all of the actions that were stored within the macro. The *WordPerfect for Windows* macros work much more logically and record the end results of a series of keystrokes. That means that you can write your macros in various ways. What matters is the endpoint of the macro.

TIP AND TRAPS FOR *WORD FOR WINDOWS* (MICROSOFT)

Word for Windows is a mature and very fast *Windows* wordprocessor. It has become the bestselling *Windows* wordprocessor and combines ease of use with considerable power. It matches the features contained in *WordPerfect for Windows* – the program that it is most frequently compared with. *Word for Windows* is the wordprocessor that 'feels' most like a *Windows* program and makes most use of the common *Windows* conventions of layout. This is probably because it has been produced by the company that developed *Windows* itself.

Word for Windows is currently available in version 6.0. It is a comprehensive program which includes charting and drawing facilities alongside the more traditional wordprocessing features. It has been made even more flexible in its latest reincarnation. The right hand mouse button can be used to edit text and paragraphs at the cursor. This saves having to use the menus or even the button bar at the top of the screen.

Another feature anticipates the common errors that you make and corrects them for you as you type. For example, I often mistype 'suprise' and 'recieve'. *Word's Autocorrect* feature allows these to be changed automatically. Apparently, Microsoft were working on the idea of this feature including the whole of the dictionary from the spell checker so that all words could be corrected 'on the fly'. Clearly, though, the memory overheads involved in such a project made this impractical. As it stands, this customizable auto-spell checker makes life a lot easier.

As with the other large scale *Windows* wordprocessors, *Word for Windows 6.0* is almost infinitely capable of being modified to suit the way you work. The tool bar at the top of the screen can hold more than one row of icons and it can be placed at the top, bottom or sides of the screen or it can be allowed to 'float' and moved to any part of the working area. Menu items can also be customized, removed or added to.

Tip

You can monitor the time you spend working on documents.

A useful feature of *Word for Windows* is the ability to keep an eye not only on the number of words in a document but also the time that you have been working on it. On the edit menu, there is a Summary Info option. Click on that and then click on the button marked Statistics. All sorts of data about the file you are working on are stored here, including the number of 'edits' you have made and the cumulative total of the amount of time that you have spent working on the document (see also the next section).

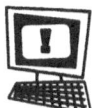

Trap

There is a word counter in *Word for Windows 2.0* but you have to search for it.

The word counting feature is buried in a menu called Summary Info which is in the file menu listing. When yo click on Summary Info a screen comes up which lists details of the name of your document and the author of it. To the right of that screen is a button which reads Statistics. Pressing this button will reveal, among lots of other things, the number of words in your current document.

Tip

Double clicking on 'empty' parts of the tool bar, ribbon and ruler offers quick access to various menus.

If you double click the left hand mouse button on a space between icons on the tool bar, you call up the options menu that allows you to customize various aspects of *Word for Windows*. If you double click on the tool bar, you call up the character menu which allows you to modify your fonts or typefaces in various ways. If you double click on the upper half of the ruler, you call up the paragraph menu which enables you to format paragraphs and if you double click on the lower half of the ruler, you call up tabs menu which allows you to customize your tab settings. Using all of these shortcuts can save time.

Tip

Double clicking on the status bar offers another menu.

If you double click the left hand mouse button on the status bar (at the bottom of the screen) you are offered the Go To menu. This allows you to jump to another page or a predetermined 'bookmark'.

Tip

Customize the Zoom 100% button.

The tool bar buttons provide the three most common levels of magnification of your document. You can customize the Zoom 100% button and then click the button with a mouse to quickly select any level of magnification from 25% to 200%.

To customize the Zoom 100% button follow these steps:

1. create a new document based on the normal template;
2. from the tools menu, choose Options;
3. in the Category box, select Tool bar;
4. in the Tool To Change box, select ViewZoom100;
5. in the Commands box, select View Zoom;
6. choose the Change button;
7. choose the Close button.

When you click the Zoom 100% button on the tool bar, *Word* displays a big arrow. As you drag down the arrow with the mouse, *Word* displays percentages from 25% to 200% in the box below the graphical arrow. To display your document at the percentage you want, release the left hand mouse button.

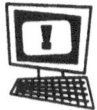

Trap

Go to top of document before you spell check.

Word for Windows, unlike some other wordprocessors, begins the spell checking process from wherever you are in a document. If you want to save a little time, go to the top of the document before you start the spell checker.

Tip

Type your text first, make your document changes later.

If you are designing a document with lots of different typefaces or margin changes, first type in all the text. When you have typed the whole document, go back and select the sections of text that you want to modify. Working this way is quicker than stopping to make changes as you go.

Tip

You can work faster in draft mode.

If you want to speed things up a little, go to the view menu and select the Draft option. This will mean that you cannot see various types of formatting such as bold and italics but it does mean that you can work more quickly through your document. This is quite useful if you are editing a document as the draft mode is surprisingly clear. On the other hand, the speed advantage gained is really only slight on a fast computer.

Tip

You can modify almost everything in *Word for Windows*.

You can set up *Word for Windows* to look and operate exactly as you want it to. You can, for example, edit the pull-down menus. You can remove certain functions from the pull-down lists or you can add your own items. You can also edit and modify the tool bar that runs along the top of the screen and you can also customize the look of the screen to a considerable extent.

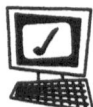

Tip

Use the Note-It function to leave yourself notes.

Note-it is a barely documented function of *Word for Windows* and one that is rarely mentioned in books about the program. You can use a variety of post-it type notes in your documents. Finding the Note-it feature is not exactly an intuitive process. You will find it in the insert menu under the Object menu item. From the menu that pops up, select Note-it and follow the instructions on the screen. You can use yellow Post-it type stickers, 'thought balloons', folders and a variety of other graphics in which to leave yourself notes in a document. Note-It works independently of the Annotation function, which is another way of leaving yourself (and others) notes in a document. Annotation is also on the insert menu.

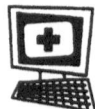

Help

Making sense of the readability indexes used by *Word for Windows*.

When you finish a grammar check of your document, you are offered a series of readability statistics, including the numbers of words, characters, paragraphs and sentences used in the document. Also included, amongst others, are the Flesch Reading Ease and the Flesch Grade Level scores. Table 7.1 helps you to make sense of those scores.

Table 7.1

Flesch reading ease	Flesch grade level	
90–100	4	Very easy
80–90	5	Easy
70–80	6	Fairly easy
60–70	7–8	Standard
50–60	9–10	Fairly difficult
30–50	11–14	Difficult
0–30	15–17	Very difficult

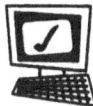

Tip

Remember that you can have more than one document open at once.

You can have up to nine documents 'open' on the screen at any one time. Be careful, though, it can become confusing if you open more than one or two. Switch to other open documents via the window menu option at the top of the screen.

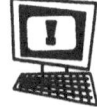

Trap

Don't try to cram too many buttons on the tool bar.

If you try to modify the tool bar too much, your buttons will disappear off the edge of the screen.

Tip

Store frequently used names and addresses.

If you use *Word for Windows* for writing letters, you can store all your most frequently used names and addresses in the Glossary feature. After you have typed a given name and address, select it by holding down the left hand mouse button and dragging the cursor over the name and address. Then select Glossary from the edit menu. 'Name' the glossary item and then select Define. Next time you need to use that name and address you can simply select it from the Glossary listing. This process becomes even easier if you link the Glossary feature to a tool bar icon. Then, if you need a name and address, all you have to do is click on the appropriate tool bar item to obtain a list of the names and addresses stored in your Glossary. You can then select the name and address that you require. Remember, too, that you can store all sorts of pieces of text in the Glossary, even boxes and diagrams.

Tip

You can customize the menu bar to add instructions to other people.

If you employ a new secretary, a research assistant, a clerical worker or anyone else who helps you with your projects, consider adding more items to the help menu at the top of the screen. This is done through the tools menu, under the Options entry. You scroll down to the menus item on that entry and enter new instructions. I have found it useful to add the following items (which trigger macros that bring information sheets to the screen) in my work in organizing a range of health care Masters degree courses:

- Who's who (a list of the people in the university college and a short note about what they do);
- MSc phone enquiries (what to do when someone phones up about the MSc courses);
- MSc applications (how applications for the MSc courses are pro- cessed) and so on.

These sit in their own section at the bottom of the help menu at the top of the screen and can be called up at any time a secretary needs details and further information. This system could easily be adapted for use in other health care settings.

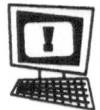

Trap

Don't remove your floppy!

If you are working on a document that is called up from a floppy disk (in A: drive), do not remove the floppy disk before working on files from your hard disk. Doing this can cause the program to crash. To be on the safe side, save your document to A: drive, close the program and restart it again before working on other files from your hard disk. This is a bug in the program that does not appear to have been fixed even in the later versions.

Tip

Select, then edit.

An important concept in working with *Word for Windows* is that things work much better if you block sections of text and then add the com- mands that change that block of text. If, for example, you want to insert bullets in front of a list of items, type the list first, then block the text and then press the bullets button. This is the other way round in *WordPerfect for Windows* where you usually select your bullet style, then type the text.

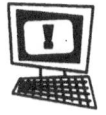

Take care with the Save button.

As with many of the *Windows* wordprocessors, if you press the Save to Disk button, there will be no warning menus to tell you that you may be writing over a previous file. Imagine for example that you have used the Letters template to produce a letter. If you press the Save to Disk button, your letter is automatically saved intact to the Letters template. That means that every time you call up the Letters template you will be presented with the full letter that you produced last time! This is clearly not what you want to happen. If you want to save a document produced with a template, always use the Save As feature, which asks you for a new name for your document.

TIPS AND TRAPS FOR *AMIPRO* FOR *WINDOWS* (LOTUS)

AmiPro is another *Windows* wordprocessor with a huge array of features. It has been extremely well thought out and is very easy to use. It can be customized very easily and you can make it look like *Word* or *WordPerfect for Windows* if you so choose. In its own right, however, it is a very versatile product that will be all many health care professionals need to manage their documents.

AmiPro can offer all of the features expected of a wordprocessor: cut and paste, spell checking, word counting and complete control over layout of documents. Much more, though, it offers a wide range of features that make it more than just a wordprocessor: *AmiPro* is a document processor. This is not just a program for writing letters but one which can produce professional reports, help you to develop forms and questionnaires and enable you to illustrate presentations.

The main opening screen is easy to understand. It offers a series of pull-down menus and also a bar of buttons across the screen made up of what Lotus calls Smarticons. Press one of these and you save your document. Press another and you spell check. Press a third and you are taken into the built-in drawing program. The range of Smarticons is almost infinitely customizable. If you don't like the range on offer, change them to suit the way you work. You can even develop your own.

Those switching to *AmiPro* from *WordPerfect* will not be disadvantaged. The program comes with a SwithchKit which shows you how to perform functions in *AmiPro* when you type in *WordPerfect* commands. This makes learning the program a straightforward and even enjoyable process. Also, Lotus use the same interface across the range of their products. Once you have learned *AmiPro* you will find the spreadsheet program *1-2-3* or *Freelance Graphics for Windows* easy to use.

AmiPro is an attractive, fast and easy to use *Windows* product. It is ideally suited to the business and management user. It comes complete with a huge range of ready-to-use templates for letters, memos, reports, slides and other business documents. It even comes with a quick-start, on-screen tutorial and an excellent manual. This is the program for the person who needs one program to do almost everything. It is also for the person who is in a hurry: *AmiPro* takes very little time to learn.

If you are thinking of changing to *Windows* and haven't yet chosen a wordprocessor, you won't be disappointed with *AmiPro* and its across-product compatibility makes it an attractive buy for the manager who is also looking for a spreadsheet, database and organizer program. For that user, Lotus offer their *SmartSuite: AmiPro, 1-2-3, Freelance Graphics for Windows, Lotus Mail* and Organizer all in one bundle.

Tip

Convert documents from other wordprocessors directly into *AmiPro*.

AmiPro does not ask you to *convert* files from other wordprocessors – it does the conversion for you. You simply open up the document in the normal way and *AmiPro* puts the file into the *AmiPro* format.

Tip

Consider using style sheets to format your work.

AmiPro comes complete with more than 55 style sheets – preformatted layouts for documents. These range from a layout for an article through various business letter formats to memo and fax sheets. You are prompted to choose between the default 'plain' style sheet or one of the 55+ templates when you start a new document. You can also edit the templates to suit your own needs.

Tip

Use the Notes feature to insert comments and reminders.

A very neat feature in *AmiPro* is that it allows you to create the computer equivalent of Post-It notes as you work on the screen. By pressing the appropriate Smarticon or button at the top of the screen, you can call up a Note, fill it in, close it and it remains embedded in your document. A small yellow square appears on the screen indicated where your Note is. This is particularly useful if you need to edit a longer document and want to leave yourself real notes. You can, of course, remove the Note whenever you want to or edit or add to it.

Tip

Use the *Adobe Font Manager*.

AmiPro comes complete with *Adobe Font Manager* which enables you to load and unload fonts as you need them. If you install lots of fonts at the same time, you slow down the running of your *Windows* applications. By allowing you to be selective about what fonts you use, *Adobe Font Manager* can speed up your way of working.

Tip

Turn off the *Windows* Print Manager.

AmiPro comes with its own print managing function and allows you to print 'in the background'. This is usually faster than working with *Windows'* own Print Manager. While you are recommended to use the *Windows* Print Manager with most programs, with *AmiPro* you are better off working with the dedicated printer function.

Tip

Use the right hand mouse button for formatting.

Like a number of database and spreadsheet programs, AmiPro makes excellent use of the right hand button of the mouse. Pressing the right hand button in a document gives you access to a wide range of document formatting functions. You can save a lot of time working in this way.

Tip

Learn the macro language.

AmiPro has an extensive macro – or 'shorthand' – facility. The program not only has macro features but offers a comprehensive programming language of its own that can enable you to customize almost all of the functions of *AmiPro*. There is on-line help in the form of a 600 page hypertext reference document on the help menu that guides you through the whole process of developing macros and using the programming language.

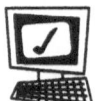

Tip

Use the SwitchKit if you are changing from *WordPerfect*.

SwitchKit – an application within *AmiPro* – will help you to learn more about *AmiPro* if you are switching from *WordPerfect*. The SwitchKit can be turned on from the help menu.

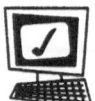

Tip

You can install a laptop version of *AmiPro*.

You can choose to install a minimal amount of the program for use on a laptop or notebook computer. This means that you do not risk erasing necessary files when trying to 'trim down' the program. Instead, *AmiPro* does the work for you.

Tip

Lotus programs make use of a common user interface.

Once you are familiar with the layout of *AmiPro* you can transfer your skills to other Lotus programs such as *Improve* or *Approach*. Lotus use a 'common look and feel' approach across their product range.

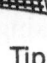

Tip

Devise your own Smarticon bars.

Smarticon is Lotus' name for the small buttons at the top of the screen which trigger commands. You can edit or develop your own Smarticon bars containing a variety of function buttons to suit the projects you are working on. Alternatively, you may find that one of the ready-made

Smarticon bars is useful. There are bars for long documents, for working with tables and for a variety of other purposes.

Tip

Lotus offer a range of macros for *AmiPro*.

Lotus has developed many macro applications in addition to the considerable range offered with the program. These macros are available through the Lotus TechLine bulletin board by calling 404-395-7707 (9600, 8 N 1) or via the Lotus WP Forum on CompuServe Information Systems. For information on the Macro Developers Kit, contact Lotus Word Processing Division.

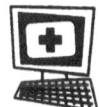

Help

Which is the best *Windows* wordprocessor?

This is a question often debated in the computing press and which creates a lot of argument in computing circles. As always with questions of this sort, there is no obvious answer. Here, for what it is worth, is my subjective opinion of the three excellent wordprocessors featured above.

First, I think that they are the best three *Windows* wordprocessors available at the moment. Although others are available, these three are the most fully featured and easy to use.

I find that *Word for Windows* is the most stable and most 'professional' in look and feel. It uses all the *Windows* conventions but this is hardly surprising given that it is published by Microsoft who also publish *Windows* itself. It is also the fastest of the three.

WordPerfect for Windows has the most features and is in many ways the easiest to use. It does a number of things better than *Word for Windows*. For example, its sorting feature is more sophisticated and it has a better master documents feature. On the other hand, it is slower and a bit 'clunkier' than *Word for Windows*. *WordPerfect* user support, though, is the best in the business. Also, the quality of the manuals is high.

AmiPro is the 'friendliest' and, in many ways, the pleasantest wordprocessor in this group. It is very easy to use and very easy to customize through its use of Smarticons. In many reports, it has come out as the 'top' wordprocessor but it has to be said that all three companies claim that their program is top of the charts, which is hardly surprising.

I used *WordPerfect for DOS* for a number of years and this is still, by far, the best DOS wordprocessor available. If you cannot run *Windows* or you choose not to, this is the wordprocessor to buy. It is very fast and has very comprehensive features. For a while, I then used *WordPerfect for Windows* and found it very comprehensive and useful. I finally switched to *Word for Windows* for its speed and for the 'way it works' – a very subjective way of evaluating a product but, in the end, an important one.

On and off, in various circumstances, I have used all three of the above *Windows* wordprocessors and if I was forced to use any of them, I would be quite happy to do so.

RECOMMENDED READING

Wyatt, A.L. (1993) *1001 Word for Windows Tips*, Jamsa Press. Available from Computer Manuals, 50 James Road, Tyseley, Birmingham B11 2BA. Telephone: 021-706-1188

Word for Windows continues to be one of the bestselling *Windows* word-processors. Jamsa Press continues its tradition of producing easy-to-use 'tips' books with this one about all aspects of working with this fully featured programs. Just to find 1001 tips is a considerable undertaking and there is little padding in this book. All of the tips are grouped under clear and logical headings: general, files, editing, formatting, styles, templates and so on. The tips range from those that will be useful to the person coming to *Word* for the first time to those for the regular or 'power' user. The format of the book means that you can soom find just the right information you need at the time. Many macros or shortcut keystrokes are described in the book and – a real bonus – these are also supplied on a disk that accompanies the book. This means that if you read about a macro that you would like to use – and there are many really useful ones in the book – you simply down-load that macro from the floppy disk. This book is essential for anyone who uses or plans to use *Word for Windows*. The program is so large that a book like this, that breaks down its complexity into easy stages, is a welcome addition to the user library.

Nelson, E. (1993) *I Hate WordPerfect But This Book Makes It Easy!* Que Corporation. Available from Computer Manuals, 50 James Road, Tyseley, Birmingham B11 2BA. Telephone: 021-706-1188

Bear with me – this is not as bad as it looks or sounds. In facing this book you have to work through one or two prejudices. First, the colour. The cover of the book is bright pink, with turquoise edging and big yellow lettering. If you plan to read it on the train you should arouse some interest in other passsengers. Second, the title. Can you imagine asking for it in a bookshop? 'Do you have a copy of ''I Hate WordPerfect But...''?' You have to be fairly extravert to cope with this one.

The book is one in a Que series of such books. It will address other programs and you will, presumably, be able to buy *I Hate DOS* and *I Hate Windows*. You could build up a whole library of *Hate* books.

The author claims that 'this is a book for people who don't want to read a book about WordPerfect'. It's all a bit convoluted. Presumably you do want to read such a book if you have been looking for one and have just bought this one. Essentially, the book aims at getting you used to *WordPerfect* as gently as possible and – obviously from the title – it takes a humorous approach.

First, though, a note of caution. When I received it, I wondered what version of *WordPerfect* it was for. After all, *WordPerfect* comes in a variety of formats. Apart from *WordPerfect* 5.0 and 5.1, there is version 6.0. There is also *WordPerfect for Windows* and a version for the Apple Macintosh. I searched for a few minutes but there was nothing on the cover to clarify the issue, nor was there anything in the introduction. After a fairly hefty search, I found the answer on the back of the title page, tucked away at the bottom: *I Hate WordPerfect* is based on *Word Perfect* version 5.1. This won't do. If you really are computer phobic and are looking for a book to guide you through the complexities of *WordPerfect*, you want to know straight away that you have picked up the right one. I only hope that the publishers rectify this in future reprints and the book is likely to run to many: it is excellent.

You come to this book expecting humour and, admittedly, different people's idea of what is funny varies. Sometimes, these sorts of approaches to learning about computing can be overdone and the humour seems forced and obvious. In this case, though, the author seems to have known what he was doing. It is funny without being distracting and comical enough to make the process of learning easy.

Also, the book is visually appealing. The American publishers do this sort of thing well. The pages are peppered with original cartoons, the text is laid out in readable blocks and a system of small pictures (or 'icons') is used to grab your attention. There is an icon called 'I Hate This!' for problems and likely danger zones, another called 'Tip', which is self-explanatory, another labelled 'Caution!' and one more called 'Experts Only' which contains tips for the more experienced user.

The first section of the book is a crash course in *WordPerfect* for the person who has never used the program before. This is simply and logically laid out and easy to work through to the production of a first document. Other sections take you on to formatting documents, handling files and then the more esoteric aspects of the program such as using columns, graphics and tables. The book closes with a section called the Quick and Dirty Dozens, which may be odd English but offers useful lists of dos and don'ts.

From its appearance, I thought I wasn't going to like this book at all. It looks loud, brash and overdone. Reading it, though, changed all that. It is well written, genuinely humorous and very useful. Anyone who needs to learn *WordPerfect* quickly would benefit from having it by their keyboard. My one concern is its shelf-life. Given that *WordPerfect 6.0* and *WordPerfect for Windows* are available and both, in their way, superseded *WordPerfect 5.1*, I wonder how much of a market remains for the book. On the other hand, the fact that *WordPerfect* remains the number 1 bestselling wordprocessing program suggests that there are still millions of copies of the 5.1, program being used.

8 Tips and traps in using databases

Most health professionals need to store information of one sort or another. Computers are particularly well suited to storing information because they are so quick and so literal. They can store huge amounts of information and return it to you just as quickly. Organizing information on a computer means using a database and this chapter offers a range of tips and traps about setting up and using databases.

Tip

Buy the right sort of database program.

There are two main sorts of database programs: the **flat file** and the **relational**. Although heftier tomes than this have been written about what constitutes a relational database and there are strict rules laid down about such things, the main difference between the two types can be described quite easily. A flat file database works with one file or one set of records at a time; it is like a box of index cards. A relational database is able to access a number of files or a number of sets of records. Imagine that you are working with a range of boxes of index cards, with different sorts of information stored in them and you have an idea of what a relational database can do. Flat file detabases are ideal for storing unidimensional data such as bibliographies or simple lists of staff details. However, if you need to call up data of different sorts and store data in different formats then you probably need a relational database.

In a health care college, for example, you may have a database file containing all the students' names and addresses. A second file might contain their marks and grades. A third file might contain the modules and options that they have completed. A relational database is able to draw together different pieces of data from all of these files.

Tip

Some excellent shareware database programs are available.

Shareware offers you the chance to try some excellent programs 'free' before you pay the registration charge. As we noted in the chapter on software, there are a number of companies that supply shareware programs and there are a number of shareware database programs available. *File Express* allows the user to set up to 2 billion forms and each field can contain up to 1000 characters (about 180 words). It is extremely easy to set up and use and works within DOS. The opening screen offers a menu from which you choose to set up a new database, call up an existing one, find information, produce or print out reports and do all the things that you expect to do with a database program. It is fast, efficient and simple to operate. Other shareware database programs include the following.

- *PCFile*. This is the classic shareware program and probably the first program to become shareware. It offers all the features expected of a good database program including the facility to 'paint the screen' – to customize the way that the information you store is displayed on the screen.

- *Wyndfields for Windows*. This is a powerful and easy to use database for *Windows* users. While it is not as powerful as some of its commercial counterparts it is still extensive in its features and is also a relational database (see above).

- *WAMPUM*. This is another program that is both simple to use and very powerful. It also includes the ability to import pictures and graphics into the database, a feature usually associated only with the more expensive commercial products.

- *Zephyr*. This is perhaps the most powerful and fastest shareware database program available. Although the beginner can use it, it is probably best suited to users who have had some experience of database usage or even to those who have had some programming experience. In the right hands, this represents exceptionally good value for money.

Tip

A simple, flat file database is supplied with *Windows*.

Cardfile, supplied with *Windows*, offers you an example of a flat file database. It can be used to store names and addresses or bibliographical references.

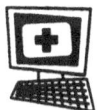

Help

Most database programs are made up of three components.

Databases not only let you store information: they allow you to access it and present it in various ways. Most database programs are made up of the following three components:

- *A design module.* The design module allows you to determine how your information will be stored in the database. Your data is stored in **forms** and **fields** and these terms are explained below. The design module is the kernel of the program and both of the other two components are linked directly to it.

- *A forms designer.* The forms designer helps you to determine how your data will be entered. Put simply, the forms designer allows you to design a form which you fill in every time you enter new information.

- *A report designer.* If the forms designer helps you to determine how information will be entered into your database, the report designer allows you to determine how the information will be presented as output. For example, from a database containing details of all the staff in a hospital, the report designer might be used to develop a listing of just the staff's names and addresses. It might also be used to develop another report which presented the staff's names and their salaries.

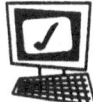

Tip

Forms and fields are key terms in most database programs.

Information in most database programs is structured in some way. In most programs this structure is achieved through the use of forms and fields. It is essential to understand these two concepts when making use of a database.

If you imagine a card file containing single cards on which are written names and addresses, each card is a **form**. A form, then, is a single but complete set of information about a particular topic.

If you pick up one of the cards in a card file, you will find that there are specific pieces of information contained on that card – perhaps the following.

- A person's name;
- That person's address;
- That person's phone number;
- Their fax number.

In database terms, each of the above pieces of information is contained within a **field**.

Surname: Brown	Department: Social Work	Fax: 453535
First Names: James David	Hospital: St Peter's	Home Phone: 356366
Identification No: DF23	Work Phone: 345245	

Figure 8.1 A form in a database program.

Surname: Brown [FIELD 1]	Department: Social Work [FIELD 4]	Fax: 453535 [FIELD 7]
First Names: James David [FIELD 2]	Hospital: St Peter's [FIELD 5]	Home Phone: 356366 [FIELD 8]
Identification No: DF23 [FIELD 3]	Work Phone: 345245 [FIELD 6]	

Figure 8.2 Fields within a form in a database program.

Thus, in summary, a database contains hundreds or thousands of forms and each form has within it fields which hold very specific pieces of information. Figures 8.1 and 8.2 illustrate the two concepts.

Tip

Read the manual before you start.

Database programs, particularly the larger ones, need to be set up properly before they can be used. If you have used wordprocessing programs, you can usually switch any one of them on and begin using the program. This is not the case with database programs. You almost always have to set up things like fields, forms and records before you start working with your database. Save yourself some frustration by spending an evening with the 'get you started' manual.

Tip

There are some excellent third-party 'how-to-use' manuals available.

Some of the larger database programs are easy to use simply but become more complicated if you want to use all of their features. Here are two examples of books that relate to the popular Paradox database programs.

Simpson, A. (1992) *Mastering Paradox 4 for DOS*, Sybex Corporation; Townsend, J.J. and Lindsay, J. (1993) *Using Paradox for Windows*, Que Corporation. Both distributed by Computer Manuals, 50 James Road, Tyseley, Birmingham B11 2BA. Telephone: 021-706-1188.

Using Paradox for Windows is one of a huge series of Que books. What is so good about these American publications is the amount of attention paid to layout and general production. They are imaginatively laid out, with plenty of 'white space' on the page. There are easy-to-digest chapters broken up by tips and screen-prints. Even though this book is nearly 800 pages long, it is not even slightly daunting. You obviously don't read it through at one sitting but, for all that, it is surprisingly readable. It is certainly more than just a reference book. You can learn *Paradox for Windows* with the help of this book. Each element of the program – and it is a huge and complex one – is broken down into short chapters. The authors clearly know the program backwards and the book is obviously authoritative. If you need not just an introduction to the program (or to others like it), the Que book and its companion volumes are worth the investment.

Paradox for Windows allows you to develop database applications in a way not seen in DOS programs. You can produce extremely professional-looking data input screens, reports and forms. You can even import pictures and illustrations. If you were keeping a database of students or staff, for example, you could keep scanned photographs of each of them with their records. None of this comes for free, however. *Paradox for Windows* takes some learning. Fortunately, Townsend and Lindsay's book makes it easier.

Mastering Paradox 4 for DOS is another example of the large scale computer publication. Like the previous volume, this is both long and comprehensive. Clearly written, it also covers all features of the DOS version of *Paradox*. It deals with installing the program, setting up database tables, searching for information, preparing reports and even with the applications feature of the program. The Applications Manager of *Paradox* allows you to build custom-made screens and to make the program work in exactly the way you want it to. You can even build stand-alone programs that give no indication at all that they originated from *Paradox*. This will be of particular interest to database developers who want to write easy-to-use programs for a variety of health care professionals. It would be possible, for instance, to build a client management program for recording primary nursing details in wards and clinics. The end user would need no prior computing knowledge as the developer (using *Paradox*) could make the whole application fit the user rather than vice versa. *Mastering Paradox 4 for DOS* explains the stages to be worked through in the Applications Manager. Using it, I built up a database system for managing courses for nursing students in five sites in about an hour. This book also explains the complexities of relational databases in simple to understand language. There are huge numbers of practical examples throughout the book and, as always, the text is well laid out.

Plan your database on paper before you switch on the computer.

Tip

Many computer database programs are quite complex and you need to plan out exactly how and what you want to store before you start the program. Do this planning with a pad of paper and a pen. This way, you can experiment with various types of layout. You can also decide what 'fields' you need and how large those fields need to be. For example, you can play around with fictitious names and addresses, count the number of letters in each of these sets of imaginary data and decide on how large your fields need to be. If you wait until you are setting up fields on your computer database program, you will find it difficult to estimate how large the various fields really need to be. In my experience, most people overestimate the amount of space they need. This uses up precious memory and hard disk space and makes opening and saving the database slower.

Tip

Find a balance.

Too many fields can take up memory and disk space, too few can mean that your database is inflexible.

Tip

Learn about 'normalization'.

Normalization is the technical term for breaking down information and data into small and discrete chunks. It is essential, if mistakes are to be avoided, that each field that you create contains only one sort of information and that no particular piece of data is stored more than once in a database system. Normalization is something of a science and an art and a considerable number of books and papers have been written about it. One of the most accessible books on the topic is Townsend, J.J. (1992) *Introduction to Databases*, Que Corporation. Understanding the basic principles of normalization is at the heart of good database design.

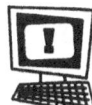

Trap

Don't break up data into fields just for the sake of it.

Most of the books on database development suggest that you should break up information into smaller chunks. For example, it is often advised that you divide up addresses into separate fields as in the following example:

Street (field 1)
Town/city (field 2)
County (field 3)
Postcode (field 4)

However, this is only important if you are going to use the data in this sort of way. For example, if you are going to want to know how many people live in a particular town, then it is essential to have 'town' as a separate field. On the other hand, if you know that you are never going to search your database in this way, you may not need to split up the information into so many fields.

A real life example of this is as follows. I set up a database to record details of the students that are enrolled in the courses that I run in a university department. At first, I used separate fields for the students' surnames, first names, street address, town name, county name and so on. Then it occurred to me that I never needed to do more than look up the students' addresses and to occasionally print them out. As I would never run complicated searches or print out parts of an address, I was able to set up a much simpler system in which the only fields I used (for this part of the database) were those of 'name' and 'address'. Consider carefully whether or not you really need to make huge numbers of divisions in your data.

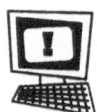

Be cautious about the amount of colour you use in database forms.

Trap

It is not uncommon for health care professionals to set up databases for other people to enter data into. If this happens, it is usual to set up a form for data entry. Modern database programs allow you to customize just about everything, including the colour schemes of such forms. When you design colour schemes for this purpose be consistent in your use of colour and also be conservative. Just because you have bright reds, blues and yellows available to you does not mean that you have to use them. Bear in mind that the person entering that data into your system may have to look at the form that you have designed everyday and, possibly, for many hours. A conservative one – and even one that makes considerable use of white, black and shades of grey – is likely to be much easier on the eye than a brightly coloured one that initially looks impressive.

Include essential instructions in a data entry form.

If you design a data entry form for a database program to be used by someone else, you can include certain entry instructions in the form. You might, for example, include details of how to save the data and how to move to the next part of the program. Alternatively, you might include instructions about the nature of the data to be entered and what must and what may be included. These sorts of instructions are particularly useful if various people have access to the data entry system of your computer.

You can use passwords for sensitive data.

Most of the larger database programs allow you to develop levels of password protection. For example, you might make a database containing datails of staff available to a variety of people at the level of names and addresses. However, you may limit access to information about salary and personal reports about staff. In this way, many people might have access at the first level, a few people at the second and only one or two people at the third. Alternatively, of course, you can protect the whole of your database system with a password. This might be important, for example, in a health care college in which student records were kept in a student database.

Norfolk (1994) offers the following list of dos and don'ts about using passwords to protect files and systems:

- don't use any names;
- don't use words which appear in dictionaries;
- don't use personal information such as a car registration number or birthday;
- don't use all digits or all the same letter;
- do include special characters;

- do use at least seven characters;
- do choose something you can type quickly.

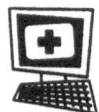

Help

Designing database systems for large organizations.

If you work in a college or a large health care organization and it has fallen to you to design a database system for the whole unit, these are the stages to work through:

- Collect all the forms that are used within the organization. These will tell you the sort of information that various people collect. Be critical of the forms and ask yourself – and the user – if they really need all the information that they ask for. Find out how that information is used and how it is filed. Also, find out how the users of that information recall it. Does it just get filed away 'just in case'? Is it entered into case notes or records? Is it fed back to students, patients or clients? All of these factors will tell you something about how to retrieve data from your database.

- Decide on whether or not you need to open up a range of files – in which case you **must** use a relational database. You might, for example, need separate tables of information for students' names and addresses, their marks over any given year, personal information and details of their previous experience and qualifications. Remember that you can recall all of this information in a single report and you can even enter all of this information through a single form. If your needs are relatively straightforward and, up until now, the information has been filed in a simple card file system, you may only need to use one file. In this case, a flat file database will meet your needs.

- Break down all of the information into discrete units. In other words, separate out names from addresses and districts from roads. You will probably find that you have very many discrete pieces of information. These will serve as guides for creating the fields in your database.

- Make sure that you have no repeating information. In other words, you should make sure that you do not have to enter the same piece of information twice. If you use multiple tables of information, it is important that you do not have to retype a person's name in each of those tables. On the other hand, to link the tables together, you must have one 'common' field in each table. Try, if you can, to use an identification number for this purpose. Don't use names to link tables together. Think about it for a moment. If you use a person's surname as the common field in a series of tables, if that person is female and gets married, you will have to change that name in all the different tables. If, however, you use an identification number, the number can stay the same even if personal details change.

- Do not collect unnecessary data. This is the principle of parsimony in form and database design. Only store information that is going to be used. On the other hand, make sure that you collect enough information. Don't trim your design back to the point where you are not storing the information that someone is likely to need.

- Once you have designed your database, hand it over to the user to try. Unless you are the person who is going to manage the database, you must make sure that users can both enter data and print out reports. Some database programs allow you to customize the look of your database to make it more user-friendly. Some even allow you to disguise the fact that they are a 'program' altogether. All the end user sees is a menu of options from which they select the functions they need.

- Be prepared to refine your data entry and report screens. However, you must stop at some point. It is easy to go on changing and refining your database beyond the point at which it continues to be cost effective to do so. Once you have finished the program and you are happy that it runs effectively, do not change it any further. Once end users have got used to the way the program works, it can be disconcerting (and a source of error) if you suddenly change the way the database operates.

- Make sure that you have built in backup facilities. Many database programs are not particularly good at encouraging you to backup your files. You **must** do this. You must backup both the program files (which contain details of how you enter and report on your data) and the data files themselves. Remember that data in a database changes frequently. Make sure that your backup system reflects this fact. This is particularly important in the health care professions in which data may concern patients or students.

Remember, too, to build in adequate levels of data protection. You must build in a password system if you are going to use the database for storing confidential information. If this is the case, check your responsibilities under the Data Protection Act. Make sure that you are allowed to store the information.

Tip

You don't have to develop the whole of your database at once.

Large databases are complicated and you shouldn't necessarily plan to finish the building of one at a single sitting. After you have set up the initial files, start by entering 'made up' data, to try out the system. If it works, key in the real data. You many find that you gradually refine the system by designing new report forms as you use the database.

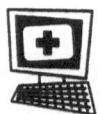

Help

An example of a relational DOS database program.

Paradox has always been a leader in the database market. The latest version, *Paradox 4*, puts it streets ahead of the competition. The name refers to the apparent paradox between the power of the program and the simplicity of use. Anyone working with it for very long will appreciate that this is, indeed, a powerful and very usable product.

Paradox 4 (Borland) is a relational database which allows you to store 'tables' of data that can be linked together in a variety of ways. Thus the principal of a health care college might open a table of information about students and then link further tables to it that contain marks, progress reports and so on. That information is then readily called up either in the form of tables or laid out in a variety of predetermined forms. In this way it is possible to view a wide range of different types of data in different sorts of ways. This is essential when comparisons are being made and contrasts are sought. Finally, data can be printed out in reports designed by the user. As if this were not enough, data can also be transferred to a range of other programs for further manipulation. Although it is not documented in the excellent and detailed manuals, I found it easy to transfer data from *Paradox* to *WordPerfect*.

Previous versions of the program have not allowed to user to use a mouse. As many people now use *Windows* as a platform for working with computer programs, the fact that *Paradox 4.0* includes a mouse facility is extremely useful. The mouse can be used to select files, manipulate data, change the size of the table in which data is being presented and for a wide range of other features. It cannot be used in all aspects of *Paradox*: it is notable, for example, that you can't use a mouse in designing report forms.

Borland have modified the look of the program and it now looks more like its sister product *Sidekick*. Also, drop-down menus have been added and this makes the selection of features very much easier. The combination of menus and the use of the mouse make this an extremely easy program to work with. Also, the new version allows you to add a memo field to your dataset. Normally, in a database of this sort, you have to decide beforehand how much data will go into any given field in the system. The inclusion of a memo field means that you can now append 'unstructured' data to a particular dataset. Thus, the college principal might want to include freeform notes about students with each entry. The memo facility allows this. It is even possible to add graphics and sound to a database.

For the everyday user, this may be the extent to which the program is used. For the more experienced user and for the program developer, there is a host of more advanced features including a whole suite of application development tools. Thus the expert might develop a custom-built database program especially tailored for the needs of a particular health care or educational organization. *Paradox* application language has become something of a standard in the database world. As with previous versions, *Paradox* is supplied with a range of well-written manuals, from a *Getting Started* book to detailed handbooks about programming.

Paradox 4.0 is likely to appeal to users at all levels, from those setting up a simple names and addresses list to managers keeping track of patients, admissions, transfers and costings. The researcher will also find it a useful analysis tool.

The new version of *Paradox* will run under *Windows* (although it is not itself a *Windows* program – Borland also produces *Paradox for Windows*). It does, however, need a more powerful computer and more memory than previous versions. It will run on 286 PCs and above with a minimum of 2Mb of RAM. It is compatible with all versions of DOS from 3.1 onwards.

Any health care manager, educator or researcher who needs to keep information in a structured format and wants to access that information quickly and easily will appreciate the speed and power of *Paradox*. It is hard to imagine any DOS database program that could compete with it.

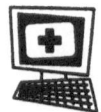

Help

An example of a relational *Windows* database program.

The *Paradox* range of database programs has rapidly developed into a market leader. The name is supposed to reflect the apparent paradox between the complexity and sophistication of the program and its ease of use. While this has been true of previous versions, it is slightly less so of this major rewrite. *Paradox for Windows* (Borland) is the *Windows* version of the database program and, obviously, you will have to be running *Windows* to use it. Also, you will have to have plenty of computer memory. At least 4 megabytes is recommended but in practice, if you want to multitask (run more than one program at the same time), 8 megabytes is a reasonable minimum.

Having mentioned those reservations, it has to be said that *Paradox for Windows* is by far the most sophisticated and powerful database program that I have used. It is also one of the most attractive. The fact that it is a *Windows* program means that it can be customized in many ways. You can change the layout on the screen, the colour schemes, the font sizes, the report functions and so on. It seems likely that you will be able to produce any form of custom-built application that you need. You will also be able to review and report on your data in just the form that you want. None of this comes, though, without a little work.

Paradox for Windows is rather different in layout from the other *Paradox* programs. It should be noted that *Paradox 4.0 for DOS* has also been released recently and if you are already using *Paradox*, this may be an attractive version too. It has been reviewed on p 146. The rewriting of the program in a *Windows* format has meant that some relearning is involved. The opening screen of the *Windows* version is quite different from the DOS version and some functions have been renamed. The relearning is worth the work.

The new program allows you to write colourful and comprehensive data entry tables. You can view these either in 'table' format or as a series of 'forms'. In the table format, you see a list of your data displayed down the screen. In the forms layout, you see one set of your data at a time, rather in the way that you might look at a series of cards.

You can produce a variety of report forms so that you can print out sets and subsets of your data and these, again, can be customized to suit your exact needs. This aspect of the program is much more comprehensive than previous versions. You can also export your data in a variety of formats and create 'dynamic links' with *Quattro*, Borland's spreadsheet program. Indeed, the two programs together offer a comprehensive range of tools for working with both textual and numerical data. It should be noted that Borland offer an *Office* package made up of *QuattroPro for Windows*, *Paradox for Windows* and *WordPerfect for Windows*. This represents both excellent value for money and the chance to buy three 'heavyweight' and comprehensive programs at once. It is unlikely that you are often going to need any other programs if you have these three and all are state-of-the-art. Also, they can each be linked to the other.

Paradox for Windows offers you various ways of working with your data. You can open up a series of 'folders', which contain series of databases. You might, for instance, keep all the details of a set of college students in one year in one 'folder' and all the students in the next year in another. In this way, you can quickly and easily organize subsets of information. Also, the use of colour means that you can colour-code sets of data. This may sound excessive but if you are dealing with a number of different databases, this immediately recognizable way of working can save a lot of time. You can also run simple and complex searches on your datasets. The 'ask' facility of previous versions of *Paradox* is now called the query function. It works in much the same way. You tick the columns that you want to search or type in examples of things that you are looking for and the program finds every instance of it. This 'query by example' approach to querying databases is intuitive and very easily learnt.

This program is likely to appeal to many different sorts of users. Health care educators will be able to use it to establish and maintain student records. I have used *Paradox* for some time now to co-ordinate a range of courses on five sites. Its simplicity and power mean that looking up student records in any one of the sites is easy and quick. Health care managers will find it useful for other sorts of record keeping and for preparing a wide range of reports. Researchers will appreciate that it can be used to store both numerical and textual data. I have known the program to be used in both quantitative and qualitative studies both as a means of storing data and also as an analysis tool. It is one of those programs that, once learned, suggests itself for use in any number of different settings.

Given the fact that some great deals are available on this product if you search through the computer magazines and that it is available as part of the Borland *Office* suite, you should consider *Paradox for Windows* as a priority if you are looking for a comprehensive database system. If you are happy working with *Windows*, you won't have too much trouble in learning how to use it. If you do not use *Windows* or do not have the time to invest in learning how to use it, *Paradox 4.0 for DOS* may suit you better. One or other of these programs is likely to be just what you need to organize your work.

Tip

Make sure you backup your database data files.

It is essential to develop a backup system for the data files contained in your database system. Database information can be some of the most important on your computer. Paradoxically, many database programs do not have particularly good systems for backing up that data. Make sure that you know exactly how to backup the files containing your information and use that backup system daily. The *program* files may or may not have to be backed up. If you have not changed the way in which the program works to any degree, you may be able to rely on the original disks for reinstalling the program if a hard disk crash occurs. On the other hand, if you have customized the program to a considerable degree – and this is likely in a large and complex database system – you must backup all of the database files: the data and the program files.

Tip

Databases can be used as educational tools.

It is possible to develop databases containing educational information about various health care topics. Students may then browse through these databases to identify specific information that they need for a project. In a study of nursing students using databases in an American college for the purpose of exploring aspects of parent–child nursing, Glazer (in Arnold and Pearson, 1992) found that students identified various advantages and disadvantages in using databases to access information. Amongst others, the students listed the following advantages:

- synthesize data faster than by pencil;
- can perform calculations;
- can form researchable questions;
- gives more global picture and enables one to look at multiple forms of data at the same time;
- able to sort, search and grade data as needed; can sift through data not needed;
- can make changes as often as needed and rearrange data with minimal work;
- can focus on data one is interested in at any given time;
- all data are in one place and not scattered on many pieces of paper;
- everyone uses the same language, which allows a mutual understanding of information;
- data can be networked and worked on by a number of people at the same time;
- decreases the need for writing and record keeping;
- content can be displayed in a wide variety of formats; can be helpful in presentation of data to prove or disprove a point, argument or hypothesis;
- can be maintained over a long period of time to reflect a historical perspective.

On the other hand, Glazer's students identified the following disadvantages of using computerized, information-centred databases.

- Frustration when unfamiliar with computers or databases.
- Time to learn how to use the computer or database was limited.
- There were limits on how the data could be entered and students had to keep looking at the manual for help.

- There was the fear of inadvertently losing data.
- The ability to retrieve data was dependent upon the data that were entered.

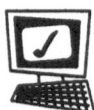

Tip

A freeform database program can be useful for handling data that does not fit into neat categories.

Researchers, managers and students often have to work with information that needs to be stored but which does not readily fall into neat categories. Researchers, for example, often battle to keep records of memos, interview transcripts and category systems, all of which fall under the heading of 'unstructured data'. Such information does not lend itself to being put into one of the mainstream database programs. Instead, an answer presents itself in the extremely useful *Idealist* (Blackwell Software).

Idealist is a program that is hard to categorize. It falls between the 'text retrieval' category and the 'freeform database'. It is wonderfully flexible and extremely easy to use.

Imagine, for example, that you want to store names and addresses, short and lengthy memos and interview transcripts all in the one file and retrieve information from that file quickly. *Idealist* allows you – with the minimum of fuss – to set up 'records' of various sorts, into which you enter your data. What marks this program out from other database programs is that almost no restriction is placed on how much data you can enter into one of those records or within the fields that you place in each record. Also, you can mix different sorts of records. Thus, you might enter a name and address as one 'record' and follow that with a full interview transcript as a 'record'. If you change your mind about the format of any particular record you simply change it to suit your needs.

What is particularly impressive is that every word entered into the database is indexed. This gives both rapid and extensive searching facilities. It also means that *Idealist* is going to be of great value to the qualitative researcher who has to make sense of huge amounts of highly differentiated data. Searching facilities include almost instantaneous 'cross-referencing' to records that contain identified words or phrases.

As with many *Windows* programs, *Idealist* can be almost infinitely customized to suit the user's needs. I managed to make the tool bar at the top of the screen match almost exactly the tool bar of *WordforWindows*. This type of customizing helps to ensure that all of the programs you use have a similar user interface and makes them even easier to use. Not that you need much help with *Idealist*. It is both intuitive and easy to use and extremely powerful. It will be of immense value in colleges and departments where unstructured data needs to be stored on computer.

RECOMMENDED READING

Townsend, J.J. (1992) *Introduction to Databases*, Que Corporation. Available from Computer Manuals, 50 James Road, Tyseley, Birmingham B11 2BA. Telephone: 021-706-1188

After wordprocessing, database programs are one of the most frequently used programs on the PC. Most health care professionals are likely to need a database for something. The researcher might keep her references on one and, sometimes, her research data. They can be used to analyse as well as store research datasets. Managers are likely to use them to store details of patients, staff, off-duty and a 1001 other pieces of information. Educators will find them indispensable for keeping track of students and their marks.

These days, database programs are easy to set up and use. *Windows* programs, in particular, are often powerful and able to produce reports of data that match the output from top-level wordprocessing programs.

What is less easy to sort out is how to plan a database system. This is where Townsend's *Introduction to Databases* is so useful. This is not a book about specific programs, nor does it tell you how to program or develop your own databases using particular programs. Instead, it offers a detailed account of how to plan your database.

One of the first rules of database organization involves what is known as **normalization**. In a nutshell, this involves breaking down the information you have into separate units and tables – subsets of the whole dataset. At first glance, this seems easy. After all, you will need a separate field for a person's name, another for their address, one for their phone number, another range of fields for the courses they study and so on. In practice, though, it becomes more complicated. If you only allow one field for an address, how will you quickly track down all the people that live in a particular town? If you allocate a number of database fields to the courses that people study, how do you account for the student who takes more than the usual number? And so on. You need to get database planning right straightaway. You cannot wait until you have entered all your data to find an important flaw in the system. Normalization involves a set of simple and straightforward rules that encourage you to think logically about your database.

Introduction to Databases is well written and full of practical, 'real-world' examples. It helps you to decide on the sort of database to buy and it also illustrates the pitfalls of buying a system too elaborate for simple needs. It highlights, too, the need for corporate planning of databases that are to be used within an organization. A chapter is devoted to the process of facilitating a planning meeting to develop a large scale database.

9 Tips and traps in writing and designing documents with a computer

Writing, like any other skill, is learned. You can learn to do it better. Many academic health professionals, like lots of other academics, write very badly. They use laboured language and convoluted sentence construction. Personal computers offer the chance to edit, edit and edit. You no longer have to rewrite from scratch – you can always change what you have written. this, of course, can also lead to weak prose. You can polish for too long. This chapter is about writing in the health professions and about making use of the personal computer in this domain. It is also about designing professional-looking documents with the help of desktop publishing and other programs.

Tip

Consider using a 'report writing' program.

As health care trusts and new educational establishments develop corporate images, the need for reports and documents of fit to 'house style' is increasingly important. *Report Styler* is a program for helping you to turn data from various sources into professional-looking documents.

Billed as 'The Desktop Publishing Program that makes your existing reports look great!' *Report Styler* (Alpha Software Corporation) fulfils some of the functions of a desktop publishing program and some of those of a top-level wordprocessor. Its great advantage is that it can draw in files from various formats, including *DBase 111* and *Paradox 111*. What it does not seem to do so easily is work with later versions of these programs. I tried, unsuccessfully, to get the program to read *Paradox 4 for DOS* files and was told by the company that I had first to convert them into *DBase 111* files. Not only is this impossible, as *DBase*

111 files are limited in the way in which they let you label data fields, but even if it were possible, it seems like a cumbersome way of doing things. I gave up on this one.

The handbook that comes with the program is excellent and includes a variety of easy-to-follow tutorials which take you through the range of things that can be done with *Report Styler*. I would like to have seen a summary of the program's capabilities at the front of the manual and a more general introduction to the program. Also, there appears not to be a section about 'error messages' and as I got some peculiar ones when trying to import files, I would have found such a section useful.

Once you have imported a file into the program, you can change almost any of its features. You can resize and replace the heading. You can change font sizes both selectively and generally. You can add new text and even import illustrations to jazz up your report. You can also reorganize columns of text in various ways and if you have ever used a desktop publishing program you will find this program easy to use.

One of the big advantages of *Report Styler* is that it allows you to set up templates for future reports. In this way, you could build a library of reports to suit a range of occasions. If you worked in a health care college, for example, you might have a similar form of report for all your mark sheets, all your student reports and all your curriculum documents. *Report Styler* allows you to develop a house style and then stick to it if you so choose. You can, of course, make any fine adjustments you like at a later date.

The big question is this: is this program going to do anything that your wordprocessor or desktop publishing program cannot do? The answer is probably yes. The fact that it can read in files from databases and spreadsheets means that you can keep a familiar format to all your documents across a range of programs. In the past, if you printed out a document from DBase it was inclined to look very different from one that emanated from *WordPerfect*. This sort of flexibility is both useful and practical.

For all that, I have worries about the compatibilities issues with up-to-date versions of database programs. *DBase and Paradox* are both in version 4 and *Report Styler* doesn't seem terribly happy reading files produced by them. On the other hand, if you have become an established user of earlier versions, then this program may be just what you need to smarten up your corporate image.

The program comes supplied on two disk sizes, is attractively packaged and very easy to install. As suggested above, the manual is useful and well designed. If you are prepared to work at the relatively easy task of learning this program you should find that your standard computer output looks more and more attractive.

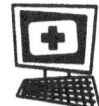

Help

Know the typesetting terminology.

Once you begin to work with various typefaces (or fonts) it is useful to know some of the basic terms that are used in typesetting. This sort of information is often useful when reading computer manuals and is even more so if you need to have your documents printed by a third-party agency. Gookin (1993) offers the following set of useful definitions:

- **Fixed.** A font in which all the characters take up the same amount of horizontal space, regardless of the actual width of the character. Examples are the Courier font in *Windows* and the text font used by MS-DOS. Compare with *Proportional*.

- **Monospaced.** Another term for *fixed* (see above).

- **Point size.** The height of the capital letter in a font, measured in points. There are 72 points in an inch, so a 36-point character is half an inch tall.

- **Proportional.** A font in which the horizontal space occupied by each character varies according to the character's width: an I takes up less space than an M. Nearly all of *Windows'* fonts are proportional and are displayed that way on the screen.

- **Sans serif.** Literally, 'without strokes'. A font with no ornamental projections or short lines hanging from its ends. These fonts are usually used in headlines because they stand out.

- **Serif.** A font with ornamental projections that extend from the ends of letters. For example, the letter T has serifs hanging from its ends like the eaves on a roof. Serif fonts are generally used for blocks of text because they're easier to read.

- **Typeface.** In traditional typesetting, each style of each font is a unique typeface: Times Roman and Times Bold are two typefaces.

In *Windows*, these two typefaces are the same font with different styles.

Consider buying extra fonts or typefaces.

If you use a computer regularly, you soon get fed up with the limited number of typefaces at your disposal. Many of the cheaper laser printers only offer a couple of fonts as standard. If you use *Windows*, this need be no problem. You simply install fonts from a disk. Ideally, you use TrueType fonts as they offer you a complete match between what you see on the screen and what you see on the printed page. Two packages, from a traditional typeface company, offer an exceptionally good range of fonts.

The wonderfully named *100 Great Faces* (Monotype Typography) is what it says: 100 classic typefaces. This is not the usual odd collection of weird and wonderful 'fancy' fonts – the sort that you sometimes find on disks given away with computer magazines. Instead, they are mixture of traditional fonts that have been used in the printing trade for years and some up-to-date faces. These are the real thing. Simply reading the list of names of the typefaces is to read something of the history of printing. Pick up a book from your bookshelf and look on the back of the title page. There, you are likely to find the name of the typeface in which the book is printed. Names like Bembo, Plantin, Garamond and Baskerville are ones that you will often come across and these are included in this package. Also included are the newspaper and 'heading' fonts such as Gill Sans and News Gothic. For the more adventurous, there is also Rockwell, a bright and brash font ideal for heading up newsletters.

Surely all this is so much pedantry? A typeface, you will say, is just a typeface. Not so. Many of the fonts that are available commercially are 'copies' of some of these original fonts (and they have odd names, to boot). Designing sets of fonts is a skilled business and you can see the difference between the real thing and mere copies when you print out your document. It is good to find a collection of fonts that includes a whole range of those designed by one of the country's leading typeface makers, Eric Gill.

100 Great Faces is going to be an essential buy for anyone who is serious about presentations of any sort. For the researcher who is printing out his or her dissertation or report, Bembo or Plantin would be ideal. Searching for the right font is even more important for the person who has to supply publishers or editors with 'camera ready copy' – text that will be photographed and used directly for publication. Such text has to be very clear and well defined. You need look no further than *100 Great Faces*. It is, quite simply, the best set of fonts on the market.

Fun Fonts, as can be discerned from the name, is a different sort of package but no less useful. Like its sister package, it contains some 'classic' fonts for display and decoration. There are typefaces to head up reports, to use for making overhead projection acetates and for newsletters. There is the brilliant modern Amasis face, designed in 1990. Also included is the beautifully named Monotype Goudy Extra Bold, which dates back to 1929. Then there is a whole selection of 'art fonts'. These are made up of over 500 special characters that can be used for decoration or for making diagrams. There is a wide selection of arrows, circles, symbols and miniature pictures. All of these can be scaled up or down and are simplicity to use. Again, anyone who is designing brochures, fly sheets or newsletters will be able to make use of these.

There is no disputing the quality of these two packages. Here is a test. Print out a page of text generated by your wordprocessor or printer. Then print out a page using fonts from either of these packages. Although the *Windows* fonts will take a little longer to print out, there is no competition. The Monotype fonts always look better.

Both packages are easy to load into *Windows* and can then be accessed by any program which uses the *Windows* Print Manager. In this way, you can ensure consistency of printout between programs. This is particularly useful in colleges and departments who are keen to develop and maintain a 'corporate image.'

If you are interested in the image you project through your writing and if you want to prepare reports, letters, essays, dissertations or publications that look really professional, either of these packages will help. You need to be careful, though. Designing a well-balanced page of text is not simply a matter of using as many fonts as you can. Most authorities recommend that you use a maximum of two or three to a page of words. Although you are spoilt for choice with these packages, it is not too difficult to pick two from the range. And the effort is worth it.

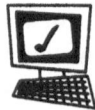

Set up a *Windows* group for managing a large writing project.

If you are writing chapters in a book or sections in a project, consider opening up a separate *Windows* group in the Program Manager. First, copy the icon of your wordprocessor to the *Windows* group. Then 'duplicate' that icon by holding down CONTROL and dragging the icon within the group. Create as many copies of the icon as you have chapters or sections. Then change the command line of each icon to fire up your wordprocessor and the relevant file. Change the description of the icon to reflect the name of the file. Here is an example.

Imagine that you have a series of files for the chapters of a book. They are called C:\book\01chap.doc, C:\book\02chap.doc and so on. Imagine that you are running *Word for Windows* as your wordprocessor. The command line for the first icon will read as follows: c:\winword\ winword.exe c:\book\01chap.doc. The command line for the second icon will read: c:\winword\winword.exe c:\book\02chap.doc. In each case, double clicking on the appropriate icon will fire up the wordprocessor and the relevant chapter of your book.

The *Windows* menu items you need for this tip are as follows. All are in the Program Manager under the file menu:

- NEW: for setting up a program group for your book or project;
- PROPERTIES: for altering the command line and the title of each icon in turn.

This process takes a little while to set up but it makes working with your larger document much quicker in the long run. I used this process during work on this book. The new program group was called Computer Book and there were *Word for Windows* icons for each of the chapters within this program group. When I want to add something to a particular chapter, I simply double clicked on the appropriate icon.

Consider using a 'dedicated' bibliographical program.

End Note Plus (Cherwell Scientific Ltd) is just such a program. All health care professionals who write essays, projects, dissertations or articles are faced with the question of how to organize references. When you first start writing, looking them up in the backs of books is no problem.

Gradually, though, it becomes obvious that you need to find some way of organizing an increasing collection of references to books, papers and other publications. Keeping a card-based system is one answer. Using a database program is another. The most flexible system that I have come across to date is *End Note Plus*. I have tried a variety of 'dedicated', computerized referencing systems but none has come close to this one. What does it do? Talking through a typical application of the program is probably the best way of describing how *End Note Plus* works in practice.

You can run the program in various ways. First, it can be run on its own as a freestanding references database program. Then, it can be used as a 'terminate and stay resident' (TSR) program that can be popped up over *WordPerfect*. Many people are likely to find this a useful way of working with it. Finally, it can be run through *Windows* and alongside a range of other programs.

This is one way of using it. Imagine that you are working on an essay or a paper in your wordprocessor. You want to support an argument with a reference but you can't quite remember the particular article or book. You call up *End Note Plus* and browse through your reference collection. Finding the right paper, you mark it, press a couple of buttons to transfer the reference to the program's 'clipboard' and then you return to your wordprocessor. You then press another couple of buttons and a note about the reference is pasted straight into your essay. So far, so good. Now comes the even more interesting bit.

When you have finished working through your essay or paper in this way, collecting references from *End Note Plus* as you work, you then have to think about how the reference list at the end of your paper will be formatted. You may, for example, want to use the Vancouver referencing system. On the other hand, the journal to which you are submitting your paper may lay down very specific instructions about how to list your references. All of this presents no problem to *End Note Plus*. At the end of your paper you simply ask the program to format your reference list in any one of a wide range of referencing styles including all the main 'academic' ones and many of the most common journal styles. In the unlikely event that your needs are not catered for, you can customize the program to produce exactly the sort of referencing style that you want.

Now imagine another scenario. You send your paper off to the journal but it is not accepted for publication. You modify it a little and then send it off to another. Before you do that, you realize that the new journal requires another style of referencing. Again, this presents no problems. *End Note Plus* allows you simply to change all of the references and your final list to suit the requirements of the second journal. In theory you could go on doing this ad infinitum.

End Note Plus offers an incredible amount of flexibility in storing, sorting, searching and organizing your reference collection. It will also generate ASCII files for transferring information to other programs and will work 'automatically' with Microsoft *Word* and *WordPerfect*. It is also fully compatible with *End Note* and *End Note Plus* on the Apple Macintosh.

Reference collections are both personal and valuable. This program not only helps you to cite references in papers and articles, it also encourages you to build your own reference library, not only of books and papers but also of computer software and other forms of 'text'. You can do simple and complex searches and build reference collections up to 32 000 entries long. It would make an ideal institutional as well as personal purchase. It comes with a very well-written manual and a large number of preset 'forms' for entering your references. If you don't like the ones you find, you can make your own. It is worth spending some time learning to use this program to its limit. It will be time well spent and will quickly be repaid by the time and energy you save when you start using the program as a writing aid.

Journals are fussy about the way in which you present your references. As a reviewer, I am still surprised by the number of writers who either do not know how to reference correctly or do not bother to check their references. This program can help you to be both consistent and accurate.

Tip

A desktop publishing program can be useful for larger or more complex writing projects.

Publisher (Microsoft) is the sort of program for people who were always nervous of desktop publishing programs. In the past, you were normally faced with a blank sheet of paper on the computer screen which you had to try to manipulate. *Publisher* still offers you that same sheet of paper but it also holds your hand as you work through the process of producing documents (or 'publications', as Microsoft would like you to call them).

On starting *Publisher*, you are invited to choose an approach to working. If you know what you are doing, you can go straight for the 'blank sheet' approach. Or you could use a template. Templates offer you preset layouts for a considerable range of business documents. One, for example, will help you to layout a brochure to publicize your organization. Others will enable you to design posters, flyers, fax cover sheets and so on. All you do is select the template and then fill in the blanks. This is the 'intermediate' starting position, perhaps for the person who has some experience of working with a desktop publishing program but not very much.

The ultimate in help, though, comes from Page Wizards. These are a particularly attractive and easy way of working. The Wizard asks you to select a particular type of document and then asks you a series of questions about that document; for example, to select the 'style' of your new creation. It then asks you for some heading text and various questions about how you would like pictures and/or text to be laid out. Finally, you just have to sit back and watch the Wizard create your document for you. This is good on a number of counts. First, it is interesting to see your document being built up in layers. Second – and more importantly – you gradually learn how to build your own documents. The Wizard is, in fact, an excellent and almost subliminal teacher.

The help does not stop there. You can choose to work with Cue Cards during your work period with the program. These are help screens that pop up on the screen to offer you tips or to make suggestions about how you might lay out the next part of your document. Once you become familiar with *Publisher*, these become annoying. No problem; you simply turn this feature off. Other help comes in the form of 'tips' that are attached to many help screens and offers of 'demonstrations'. If you make a mistake, the program asks you if you would like to be 'shown' how to do a certain operation.

It is easy to become blasé about all this. Most programs, after all, offer you help but never, in my experience, to this sort of degree. This program can be used by the absolute beginner as well as the experienced manager, educator or clinician who knows how to work with *Windows* programs. For them, almost all of the help can be turned off.

All of this works on top of an extremely powerful desktop publishing program. *Publisher* is fully featured program that allows you to manipulate text to degrees unheard off a few years ago. It enables you to create formal and less formal creations that will enhance the quality of the documents that you produce on your PC. You can import text from other programs (such as *Word for Windows*) and you can insert pictures, tables and all of the other objects that go to make up designed documents. You can lay out books and reports, newsletters and advertisements, design conference posters and flyers and develop your own corporate logos and stationery.

As always with Microsoft publications, the manual is extremely well written. It is clear that Microsoft are paying attention to what end users really need from a computer program. *Publisher* may not be the absolute top of the range in desktop publishing programs, but it is something far better: a desktop publishing program for all users.

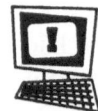

Trap

Desktop publishing can use a lot of laser printer memory.

If you use a laser printer for printing out the results of your desktop publishing, you are likely to want to use a laser printer. Bear in mind that complicated page layout means that you need lots of laser printer memory. You may want to consider 2Mb as a minimum requirement if your layouts are complicated. Remember that this is printer memory and not computer memory (RAM).

Tip

You may want to illustrate your reports using a graphics program.

There are a variety of graphics programs available for the PC but few, if any, can match *Corel DRAW!* (Corel Corporation). The statistics alone are breathtaking. *Corel DRAW!* 4.0 comes with 755 fonts, all of which are scalable. If you can't find the typeface you need amongst that lot, you are looking for the wrong one. Then there is clip art. There are 11 476 graphics images in *Corel DRAW!*'s own format, 5200 symbols, 329 paint and photograph images, 330 chart templates, 348 animation files and 420 cartoons. Altogether, the package contains more than 18 000 clip art images and symbols. In fact, all of the clip art images are printed out in their own paperback book. Everything is included – even the kitchen sink (clip art image 063).

Most users will want the package for *Corel DRAW!* itself. This is a top-level drawing and illustration program which lets you create original praphics or modify those offered in the above listings. In experienced hands, the program can help to produce top-quality illustrations. What's more, the program is easy and intuitive to use. As with all *Windows* programs, *Corel DRAW!* uses pull-down menus as well as rows of buttons at the top of the screen. Also, it makes use of 'roll up' menus. Just the top of the menu stays visible on the screen until activated. Then, a whole series of useful commands are at hand.

Corel DRAW! also has extensive desktop publishing features and can produce documents of up to 999 pages in length. Text from wordprocessors can easily be imported and then manipulated in any number of ways. Illustrations can then be inserted into the text and final productions can be as simple or as complex as you like. One of the striking features of the program – one amongst thousands – is the undo – redo feature. If you don't like a change that you have just made to text or a picture, you can 'undo' the modification. Changed your mind? Simple: you just redo the modification. In fact, there are 99 levels of 'undoing'. This means that you can construct and deconstruct images to very sophisticated degrees.

Corel DRAW! is not just one program. In the same box comes *Corel CHART!*, *Corel SHOW!*, *Corel MOVE!*, *Corel TRACE!*, *Corel PHOTO-PAINT!* and *Corel MOSAIC!*. Any one of these programs could be sold as a stand-alone, although the exclamation marks can wear you out. That they are all included in the one box makes this program excellent value. The one most likely to be of use to health care professionals in management, education and research is *Corel CHART!*. This is a spectacular charting program that allows you to produce extremely professional-looking bar charts, histograms, pie charts, etc. As we have seen, your choice is not limited. There are 80 chart styles to choose from and if you don't like any of those, you can invent your own.

Corel SHOW! allows you to make 'slides' that are shown on the computer screen. This feature would be of value to professional educators who were keen to develop their own sophisticated learning packages. *Corel TRACE!* is an unusual tracing program that helps you adapt scanned-in photographs. *Corel PHOTO-PAINT!* is an all-round painting and image manipulation package. *Corel MOVE!* helps you to make animated screen productions, while *Corel MOSAIC!* helps you to organize clip art and finished drawings. Altogether, a highly integrated and extremely comprehensive set of tools.

You can install the whole of *Corel DRAW!*, in which case you will need an incredible 45Mb of disk space, or you can simply install the parts of the program you need. Alternatively, you can run the whole thing off one of the two CD-ROMS that come with the package. These contain much more of the clip art and fonts than the disks and they also contain an excellant animated introduction to using *Corel Draw!*.

Everything is not completely rosy. Given the size of this program it is hardly surprising that there are one or two bugs in it. These can, very occasionally, cause systems crashes but while these have been reported elsewhere, I only had one such experience. I found it quite possible to produce very detailed bar charts, pie charts and diagrams without consulting the excellent manual. This 'blind' approach to new software is often a very good guide to how the program will work in everyday terms. Whilst it is clearly not a program for the absolute beginner, anyone who is familiar with basic *Windows* commands will soon find themselves producing useful work with *Corel DRAW!*.

Corel are to continue to supply *Corel DRAW!* 3 at a very much reduced price. Although this does not offer all the features of the latest version, it represents extremely good value for money.

If you need to publish articles, reports or books that contain diagrams or charts, it is usually vital that the 'roughs' you send in are almost identical to what you anticipate will appear on the printed page. After all, the editor cannot read your mind nor anticipate what you really wanted. A program like this can make sure that your 'roughs' really do match the final product. *Corel DRAW!* is also ideal for producing camera-ready copy. Many journals and publishing houses will be only too pleased to accept your artwork ready-made. But it has to be good.

If you are in the market for a graphics package that will help you to illustrate your research reports, enable you to work on figures and charts for research reports up to a publishable standard, then *Corel DRAW!* is for you. It combines simplicity of layout and ease of use with a degree of exhaustive sophistication that will take you years to grow out of. This package is exciting to work with and really can aid productivity.

Tip

If you have a modem, you can download references from on-line reference databases.

This is a useful feature for those who need to search the literature in their field on a regular basis. A modem allows you to 'communicate' with various services, from your computer, via a telephone line. It also allows you access to various on-line reference database services. Kilby and McAlindon (1992) suggest the following advantages of computer literature searching. You can:

- run literature searches at almost any time of day or night, at your convenience;
- search from a computer terminal located in the library or in your home or office (depending on the system being searched);
- conduct on-the-spot searches to respond to questions that need immediate answers;
- modify a strategy during the search if you are not finding the information you need. As a result, searches may be more on target.
- browse through the databases and build your knowledge each time you search. Literature searches are a direct form of continuing education to assist you with keeping up with trends and familiarizing yourself with a new area;
- take advantage of a wonderful opportunity for serendipitous discovery of data related to your topic;
- quickly identify pertinent literature as it is indexed (one database, Medline, is upgraded weekly);
- easily and efficiently create and update tailor-made bibliographies;
- experience a feeling of power as you realize that you have access to a vast amount of information your computer.

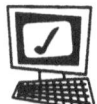

Tip

Consider using a grammar checker.

Nowadays, most of the larger *Windows* wordprocessors include a grammar checker as standard. *Grammatik for DOS* (Reference Software International) is a stand-alone grammar checking program. What does it do? It would be impossible to list all of *Grammatik's* functions.

Essentially, it is grammar checking software that proofreads word-processed documents for errors in grammar, style, usage, punctuation and spelling. It explains errors, gives advice and suggests replacements (where appropriate). It offers a useful means of avoiding jargon, complicated sentences, redundancy and excessive use of passive voice. In other words, it can help you to write clearer and more lively prose. You can also compare what you have written with different types of styles: general, business, letter, memo, report, technical, journalism and fiction to name but a few. It also compares your work with a standard business document and (for some reason) one of Churchill's speeches. You can learn a lot from this program. If you are not sure about your grammar, you will be after using *Grammatik*.

To run the full program through a long document takes time. The program works to so many rules that even a reasonably simple piece is usually taken apart at the seams. This means that the program will stop at every instance of what it conisders to be a mistake and offer you the chance to put things right. If you don't like this way of working, you can ask the program to prepare you a special list of mistakes which you can work through later. If you get called away from an editing session, you can use the 'bookmark' feature to let you come back to where you left off.

As with any style and grammar checker, it has its limitations. It is quite possible to offer it a piece of nonsense with perfect grammar and spelling and it will assure you that your nonsense is well written and easy to read. The ultimate grammar checker is some way off but until it arrives, *Grammatik* does the job well.

If you are writing for publication, respect certain conventions.

Tip

Many health professionals have to write articles, papers and book manuscripts for consideration for publication. These are a few conventions that you should observe when preparing your manuscript.

- Do not justify the right hand side of your text. Justified right text is difficult to read when there is a lot of it. Justify the left hand side of the text only.

- Double line space your manuscript.

- Make sure that all your pages are numbered consecutively.

- Make sure that your diagrams are accurate and that they look they way you want them printed. The editor or art director cannot know what you want if you only submit a rough draft.

- Avoid 'uprights' in diagrams as far as possible. If possible, limit the lines in your diagrams to horizontal ones. Vertical lines are more expensive to set.

- Make sure that you read Advice to Authors before submitting manuscripts to journals and the advice booklets that publishers produce if you are preparing a book manuscript. Follow both of them to the letter.

Tip

Use a specialist program if you need to draw organizational charts in your documents.

Many health care managers and educators find that they need to draw fairly complicated, hierarchical charts to represent their organizations or institutions. Drawing them can be difficult with an ordinary wordprocessor or even a graphics package. With *Org Plus* (Roderick Manhatten) you can model your organization either as it is or as you would like it to be. It allows you to explore the possible as well as the actual.

Once installed on your hard disk, the program is simplicity to use. The accompanying manual is very well written and describes some of the details of the program. You will have no problem, though, in finding out how the program works by simply using it. Its Windows interface means that it has a familiar look to its basic layout and works in the way that you expect it to.

Nor are you limited to straightforward, 'top-down' organizational charts. The program offers you a whole range of styles of chart and if you don't like the one that you start with, you simply change it. As can be expected, you can modify just about anything you want, after you have drawn it. You can personalize your charts by adding your own health authority's logo as *Org Plus* allows you to import 'objects'– graphical designs and pictures imported from other programs. A complete set of drawing tools lets you get special effects that can't be produced automatically by the program. Printing out your chart is simplicity itself and, I found, best done through the *Windows* Print Manager. As with most programs working through the Print Manager, *Org Plus* can access all of the fonts that you currently have available through *Windows*.

The new version of this program also supports object linking and embedding. This feature allows you to make 'live links' between a diagram or illustration in *Org Plus* and one in another program. Thus you may want to be able to modify certain elements of your charts in, say, your wordprocessing program. As you do this, your *Org Plus* chart will automatically be updated as well. This sort of flexibility and ability to link *Org Plus* with a range of wordprocessors, databases and drawing programs adds even more to its usability. The more you use object linking and embedding, the more uses you find for it. Also, it allows you to ensure a uniformity in the documents you create in various sorts of programs. This is particularly important if you are trying to develop a corporate image or you simply want to project a professional approach to document production.

Org Plus does what it does extremely well. Clearly, this is not going to be a program that every computer user uses every day. On the other hand, if you are a manager or a senior educator who needs to produce reports or curriculum documents in a hurry, this sort of program is just what you need. The fact that it is extremely easy to use makes it even more attractive.

Org Plus, despite the fact that it is marketed solely as a tool for drawing organizational charts, can also be used for other sorts of diagrams. It might be used to draw family trees and I can imagine its being useful in mapping family relationships in mental health settings. It can also be used to draw illustrations and diagrams in research reports.

The program has a very stable feel to it and is extremely well presented. It comes on two sizes of disk and the accompanying manual is straightforward, detailed and clear. As anyone who has had any experience of computer manuals will know, this is not always the case. It is hardly surprising that this has become a bestselling business program. If you are in education, research or management, you are likely to find a need for it at some time. It will make the difference between a good report or brochure and a really professional one.

RECOMMENDED READING

Parker, R.C. (1993) *Looking Good In Print: A Guide to Basic Design for Desktop Publishing*, 3rd edn, Ventana Press, North Carolina. Available from Computer Manuals, 50 James Road, Tyseley, Birmingham B11 2BA. Telephone: 021-706-1188

More and more managers and students are using personal computers for preparing work for publication or for presentation. These days, it is not sufficient to merely 'type' something. If you want to make an impression – and in these days of market pressures, most people do – then you need some help in making a visual and textual impact. This book won't turn you into a designer but it will help you to develop more professional-looking documents.

The amateur tends to overuse the special effects that can be achieved with a wordprocessor or desktop publishing program. Part of the art of achieving good results is to use restraint. *Looking Good in Print* helps you to avoid the worst excesses of computer textual design.

The book itself is a good example of what it is aiming to teach. It was laid out by the author and designed on a personal computer using a fairly widely used desktop publishing program.

Opening chapters deal with the basics of layout and design. Further chapters show you how to use 'grids' to organize your work and to achieve consistency. In this section, too, there is all sorts of advice about the use of headlines, headers and footers, styles and margin sizes. The next section covers, very extensively, the use of fonts or typefaces. Another section discusses and demonstrates the effective use of graphics and final chapters give extended examples of how to lay out specific sorts of documents, from newsletters to brochures.

This is going to be a valuable resource to many health care prof-essionals. Anyone who has tried to design a promotional booklet for their college or organization will know how difficult it is to produce top quality work. With *Looking Good in Print*, most computer users will be turning out imaginative and goodlooking documents. Highly recommended.

10 Tips and traps in using computers for research

Personal computers are particularly well suited to research work. The desktop computer can handle huge amounts of data, both numerical and textual. There are programs available to analyse all types of data. Notebook computers make it possible to collect data in the field, directly into the computer. Notebook computers today are as powerful and have as much memory and hard disk space as the largest desktops of a few years ago. Some people even use laptops as their main computers. This chapter offers some pointers in using personal computers in health related research. Both qualitative and quantitative approaches to research are addressed.

Tip

Consider using a project manager to organize larger research projects.

Developing and planning long and short term research projects used to involve graph paper and complicated wall charts. Now you can get your projects organized, much more efficiently, with a computer program. *Microsoft Project* (Microsoft) is what it says: a program for organizing all elements of any type of project. Health care professionals are likely to find it particularly useful for organizing research projects, organizational change, long term management development, trials, conferences and curriculum plans.

There are three phases to project management. First, you create the project. This is traditionally the 'brainstorming' phase. *Project* allows you to play around with possibilities and then to structure a framework for organizing the project. Second, you manage the project. *Project* allows you to keep track of all the elements of your project, predict problems, reallocate time and make all sorts of fine adjustments. Third, you produce reports of the project. Again, *Project* helps here by creating informative and attractive reports quickly and easily.

The project management techniques that *Project* offers are comprehensive. You can use the critical path method of scheduling – an approach already in use by many managers. Or you can use the program evaluation review technique (PERT) – another method that has often been used in the health care professions to organize and manage the use of time. Finally, you can use Gantt charts – perhaps the most familiar way of illustrating time spans in a project.

Initially, you can enter 'events' in your project into a spreadsheet-type screen. Then you can reorder events, retime them, reschedule them and manipulate those events to a considerable degree. Various views of your data allow you different perspectives on your project. The business of working with *Project* takes you far beyond a mere paper exercise. The program can help you develop and think through both large and small projects. Fundholders will appreciate being able to time and cost sections of projects and know that they can always run projects of the 'what if?' sort.

This is not a program to load up and work with immediately. You have to invest a little effort in getting to know it. Fortunately, as with many new Microsoft programs, a good deal of help is at hand. First, you get a run-through of the main points of the program when you first start it up. Then, you can have the program 'talk you through' the various elements of project design and scheduling. Finally, you can call up context-sensitive help at any time. Also, the reference manual is excellent and informative. Microsoft produce readable manuals. These are not simply alphabetical lists of what programs do. Instead, they are laid out in easy to follow and easy to digest chapters.

Project is highly compatible with other *Windows* programs and particularly with other Microsoft programs. If you already use *Word for Windows* or *Excel*, you will soon get used to *Project*. It uses the common user interface that runs throughout the Microsoft range of programs and honours all of the *Windows* 'conventions.'

Tip

Searching the literature.

Recent developments in technology have meant that information is more readily available than has previously been the case. We are no longer dependent only on finding reports in books and journals.

Instead, we can augment those findings through computer searches. This section outlines some of the facilities that are available to the person who wants to do a literature review.

Two methods of searching can be described: the **incremental** approach and the **broad brush** approach. The incremental approach involves carefully tracing back a variety of 'leads' to their source. The person who uses the incremental approach will find one or two key papers. They will then read those papers and note the references that **that** author cites. They then track down those papers and continue the process. In this way, a systematic searching of the literature is undertaken by a gradual and unfolding process of exploring one aspect of the field at a time. The incremental approach is a rigorous one but it can also be very time consuming. It is best suited, perhaps, to projects that are very specific, very clearly defined and in which the researcher knows that little other literature is likely to exist about the topic. The incremental approach starts, then, with the researcher finding perhaps a single paper on the topic under investigation and following through the process identified above.

Where does the researcher look for papers on any given topic? The usual advice here is to look at the 'heavyweight' and referred journals first. These will contain research reports and well argued theory papers that are appropriately referenced.

The broad brush approach to searching the literature involves the researcher amassing as many references about a particular topic as possible and then filtering through the references and choosing the ones that are particularly pertinent to the study in hand. The broad brush approach often involves having access to computer searching facilities. Increasingly, schools, colleges and university departments are investing in a CD-ROM system which involve a computer which can read compact disks. Those disks are almost identical to the ones used in the music industry except that they contain huge amounts of computer data rather than music data. They can only be 'read' by the computer and cannot be 'written to'. The CDs in this case contain bibliographies and abstracts relating to particular fields of study. A library does not simply buy one set of disks but subscribes to new issues and updates. In this way, the CD-ROM collection stays up to date and contemporary. Examples of databases available on CD-ROM include the following.

- *Medline*
- *Nursing and Allied Health Database*

- *ERIC*
- *Health Encyclopaedia*
- *Health Education Bibliography*

It is highly unlikely that any one library will subscribe to all these databases but many will subscribe to *Medline* and *Allied Health Database*.

The researcher who uses the CD-ROM system first decides on **keywords** for a search. Let us imagine that the researcher is doing research in the field of counselling in nursing. He or she has to consider what sort of words might appear in the titles of books and papers in the field. The computer will search through the bibliographies and abstracts and look for these particular words. Thus, the researcher may decide to search for everything that has 'counselling' in the title. They are likely to find that this single word is 'too big' and generates thousands of references. Fortunately, the CD-ROM program will tell you how many references have been found before it prints them out or helps you to transfer them to disk.

Having found that 'counselling' generated too many references, the researcher may find it necessary to be more specific in choosing their keywords. Thus, they may decide to use the words 'counselling and nursing' and 'counselling and psychiatric nursing'. The actual search terms used will depend on the particular researcher's needs and wants and the slant of their research program. The choice of keywords involves both creativity and a certain amount of experimentation. Often, initial searches turn up too many or too few references and it is simply a matter of adapting the search words to ensure that 'enough' references are obtained. There is no magic number here. It is impossible to say what is the 'right' number of references to turn up in a computer search. Much will depend on the size of the field, the prior knowledge that the researcher has of the extent of that field and the nature of the project being undertaken.

The CD-ROM search will, after some work, give the researcher access to a full list of references to books and papers on the topic in question. Some bibliographies published within the CD-ROM system also offer detailed abstracts of each reference. This facility can be particularly useful in deciding whether or not to obtain an offprint of the paper or chapter.

Once the program has found the list of references, the researcher has to consider whether or not they want to have that list printed (in which case they will simply send the list to the printer plugged into the computer). The alternative, however, is to have the list downloaded to a floppy disk. In this case, the researcher brings their own disk to the computer and asks the program to copy the list on the screen to their own disk. The advantage of this approach is that the researcher can then work through the list on their own computer and even copy the list of references to their own bibliographic program.

The broad brush approach to literature reviewing always leads to a huge list of references. The researcher then has to work through that list and decide which references to follow up and which to reject. The point here is that all the computer can do is select the list of references. The researcher has to make decisions about what is and what is not appropriate to the study in hand. Once a smaller list of 'musts' is obtained in this way, the researcher then has to find copies of the papers and book chapters. One way of doing this is by looking up the papers in libraries of back copies and in the local library. The other is to send off to the authors of the papers and chapters to ask for copies. Whichever approach is used, the researcher eventually ends up with a large collection of papers and chapters which then have to be read and the details recorded. There are a variety of other publications about how to search the literature.

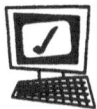

You can use one program to devise and analyse your questionnaires.

Tip

Questionnaires are notoriously difficult to develop. Once you have devised your questions, you then need to design your questionnaire. You may need another program to analyse the responses to it.

PinPoint (Longman Logotron) is an excellent program that combines almost all of the stages of the questionnaire design and analysis process. Having written your items, you design your questionnaire format. *Pin-Point* offers you a range of styles for your questionnaire items, ranging from simple 'yes/no' responses to multiple choice responses to items that require the respondent to enter text. Once you have designed your items on the page, you can customize the look of your questionnaire with a range of graphical and text editing functions. You can enter images and text and even import textual and graphical information from other programs.

Next, you can either print out copies of your questionnaire or you can invite your respondents to fill it in on the screen. This cuts out one stage of the survey process at a stroke and might be ideal if you are using a notebook computer and a fairly lengthy questionnaire.

Responses to your questionnaire items are fed back into the program once they have been returned. These can be entered either via copies of the questionnaire on the screen or via a spreadsheet-like table. The fact that the on-screen questionnaire can be used for entering results is likely to mean that errors in data entry are reduced. It also means that, in a larger health care institution, clerical or secretarial staff might be used to enter the data. The approach offers the most 'logical' approach to data entry as the image on-screen matches, exactly, the questionnaire itself.

Finally, *PinPoint* enables you to do all the usual calculations. You can quickly generate frequency counts of the responses to your questionnaire and then you can chart the findings. Various sorts of charting facilities are offered. You can print bar charts, pie charts and a range of other ways of illustrating your findings.

Usually, when you design and develop a questionnaire, you start with your wordprocessor and generate items. Then, you might use a graphics package or even a desktop publishing program to design the layout. Finally, you have to enter your findings into a statistics package or a spreadsheet program in order to analyse your findings. With some statistical packages you may then have to make another move – back to your graphics package – to draw figures and charts. *PinPoint* incorporates all of these features into one easy-to-use program. It follows all of the usual *Windows* 'conventions' in terms of the layout of the program on the screen which makes it very easy to get to grips with. It also comes with an excellent manual that talks you through the stages of development of your questionnaire and a range of sample questionnaires to give you an idea of what can be produced. All in all, an excellent program for the beginner and expert alike.

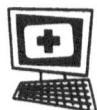

Help

Using a wordprocessor to content analyse textual data.

The analysis of data obtained from semistructured and unstructured interviews is an essential part of many qualitative research studies. The example text used in this tip is drawn from data generated in a study carried out by the author into AIDS counselling. The wordprocessor used in the study was *WordPerfect 5.1* (WordPerfect UK) but the stages described below can be worked through on any fully featured word-processing program which has cut-and-paste, sorting and searching facilities. The approach could be modified for use with wordprocessors which do not have all of these features. It will be noted that other programs are available in order to carry out this sort of analysis although these programs (such as *The Ethnograph*) are sometimes expensive and not always easy to get hold of.

Whilst the example offered is of an analysis of a series of interview transcripts, the method could easily be applied to written text as long as it was in a computer file. It may be recalled that text can nearly always be easily transferred between different wordprocessing pro-grams via ASCII files. ASCII files (American Standard Code Information Interchange) are ones that contain only essential textual codes and which can be 'read' by almost all computer programs.

The aim of content analysis of text from interview transcripts is to illustrate, through the use of headings and subheadings, all the issues that were discussed by respondents during their interviews. The method described here offers a rigorous way of grouping together themes in such a way that all the text contained in a series of interviews is accounted for. The text used in the example described below was selected from transcripts of 24 interviews conducted with nurse edu-cators, AIDS counsellors and other AIDS workers. The aim of the study from which this text was drawn was to identify the perceptions of various workers in the AIDS field regarding the work of AIDS counsellors.

During the semistructured interviews, a question that was fre-quently asked by the researcher was: 'What are the psychosocial problems of the person with AIDS?'. Review of the transcripts revealed that this question (or a slight variant of it) occurred in 18 of the 24 interviews. For the purposes of description in this tip, the text that followed that question, in the 18 cases, was cut out of the transcripts and all 18 sets of responses were placed together in a *WordPerfect* file.

The transcripts were themselves contained in *WordPerfect* files and so no further conversion of the text was necessary. Thus the raw text that was ready to be content analysed consisted of 18 responses to the above question, contained in a single textual file.

FIRST TASK

First, the block of text that contained the 18 responses was 'sentence-busted'. That is to say, by use of the 'search and replace' feature in the wordprocessing program, each sentence was separated from its counterpart and allowed to stand on a line of its own. This is achieved by replacing each full stop in the text with a full stop followed by a carriage return. The effect is to divide the text up into single sentences. A second 'search and replace' was also conducted to account for sentences that ended in a question mark. In this case, each question mark was replaced by a question mark and a carriage return. The font (or character) size of the text was then reduced on the screen and the margins on the screen narrowed in order to allow each sentence to occupy one line on the screen. An example of what this sort of text looked like is illustrated below:

> The main problem is educating the health care worker right across the board.
> Doctors in particular, counselling skills for doctors.
> Everybody needs education.

This form of 'sentence busting' made it much easier to begin to identify the themes that were 'hidden' in the text. Altogether, 216 separate sentences were identified and, thus, 216 potential items for classification. A decision had to be made about fragments of text and about odd sentences that appear out of context in this form of textual breakdown (e.g. 'This can be a problem, sometimes' or 'Other people have had this problem, too'). In almost all cases, these decontextualized sentences did not appear to add or detract from understanding the remaining sentences.

It should be borne in mind that this type of analysis can only ever work at the level of overt content: latent content cannot be addressed through analysis methods of this sort. That is to say, the analysis is a literal one of the words and phrases on the page. It cannot offer any insights into what the respondent 'might' have meant or into any 'hidden' meanings. It is arguable, anyway, whether any such attempts to 'read between the lines' are possible. Analysis aimed at latent content can only really be carried out in the presence of the respondents themselves and in negotiation with them.

Next, the sentences were worked through one at a time and further divided to ensure that each line of text only contained one item of information. For example, a sentence that read as follows:

They experience fear, depression, sometimes they don't know who to turn to . . .'

was separated thus:

They experience fear . . .
Depression . . .
They don't know who to turn to . . .

This increased the total number of items, in single lines, to 265 and this format meant that the whole of the text had been divided up into discrete units and that each unit contained a single item of information to be classified.

SECOND TASK

Next, all items were sorted alphabetically by line. This allowed for certain grouping to occur. For example, a number of the respondents began sentences or utterances with the word 'fear'. The process of alphabetical sorting allowed for all of these utterances to fall together and thus made the process of classification a little easier. This stage could be omitted if the researcher was working with a wordprocessor that did not allow for sorting in this way. Most of the larger word-processors now have such a function.

THIRD TASK

This was the most 'subjective' stage of the process. The sentence-busted text, organized alphabetically, was printed out and the process of 'open coding' was carried out. Open coding refers to the process of jotting down single words or short sentences that summarize each of the issues contained in the text. The aim was to use as few phrases as possible to capture all of the ideas expressed in the text and as many as were required to ensure that every idea was accounted for. Through a slow process of working and reworking the phrases and of cutting out repetitions, the following 17 headings were generated:

1. acceptance issues
2. fear of different sorts
3. alienation and loneliness
4. strong emotions
5. self-blame
6. health care facilities
7. who to tell
8. life insurance/benefits
9. transmission
10. stigma
11. Nemesis
12. related psychological/social issues
13. death and dying
14. gay issues
15. travelling
16. haemophiliac issues
17. the church.

These 17 headings could account for everything that had been referred to by all of the respondents. This may be rather a large number of categories to use if the researcher is working 'manually' (i.e. without the use of a computer) but the number can be catered for when using a wordprocessor. As will be noted, each of the categories was given a number.

FOURTH TASK

The next stage was to work through the sentences, allocating each a number according to the category system referred to above. Thus, sentences that related to death and dying had a number 13 typed into the left hand margin. Sentences that were about having AIDS and travelling were allocated the number 15 and so on until all of the sentences were accounted for in this way.

FIFTH TASK

Once all the sentences had been categorized in this way, the list of numbered sentences was sorted again, this time numerically and in ascending order. This process allowed *WordPerfect* to bring together all the '1's, all the '2's, all the '3's and so on. At the touch of a few buttons, the whole of the text was sorted into categories and all of the sentences allocated to a particular category were grouped together. An example of one such grouping is offered below.

10. Stigma

10. They may also feel victimized.
10. Stigmatization is the thing that they often feel.
10. There is a massive stigma attached to it.
10. People see it as related to drugs and people will think I'm a drug addict.
10. Stigmatization.
10. They think of stigma and prejudice.
10. Social stigma is the real problem.
10. There is leperization either by others or themselves.

The example above illustrates all of the items categorized '10' and the '10' category related to 'stigma'.

SIXTH TASK

Once all of the items were pulled together under each of the categories in this way, the number of items in each category could be counted. A word of caution is offered here. Little can be made of the number that is generated in this way. It cannot be assumed that, because the system of analysis produced 14 items under the heading of 'death and dying' and only two items under the heading 'travelling', 'death and dying' was a more important concept to the respondents. The production of these numbers of items may be an artefact of the categorization system which, to some degree, is arbitrary and, in any case, is produced by the researcher. What the numbers do help with is in deciding whether or not the category system is diverse enough. For example, in the first attempt at the development of the category system, a category called 'psychological issues' was produced. When the dataset was itemized, numbered and sorted, it was found that this category had 32 items in it. The next nearest category had 14 items. This suggested that the 'psychological issues' category was too 'large' and subsequently it was broken down into three smaller categories.

SEVENTH TASK

The stages described above allow the researcher to offer, in a concise format, an account of all the issues discussed under a range of headings. Before a research report describing and then accounting for these findings is written up, checks for the validity of the analysis need to be carried out. There are at least two ways in which this can be done. First, the researcher can return to respondents and check with them the degree to which they do or do not agree that the categories generated really do classify their utterances clearly and honestly. Second, the researcher may ask two colleagues (one with some experience of content analysis and the other without) to check the system or, perhaps, to generate their own independently of the researcher's original system. Such a process of validation can enable the researcher to check their own bias and can sometimes throw new light on the data.

Also, the findings need to be compared with the complete transcripts. This check is to ensure that the sentences analysed in the way described above do not misrepresent the respondents' views when those sentences are viewed in the larger context of the transcript.

It may be said that this method of analysis is probably most useful when the answers to interview questions are fairly short and fairly precise. It will be recalled that, in the case described here, respondents were asked to identify 'psychosocial problems': they usually did this fairly concisely. Clearly, a lengthy answer which involved considerable discussion and qualification would not readily lend itself to being broken down into single sentences in this way. An alternative, however, would be to divide the transcripts up into longer units, sometimes known as 'meaning units'. Usually longer than a single sentence, a meaning unit is a small extract of text which, on its own, forms a discrete and meaningful utterance.

EIGHTH TASK

Finally, the findings can be written up. When the findings are presented under the series of categories generated by the content analysis, decisions have to be made about a variety of issues. First, the researcher needs to consider whether or not to link each category to the literature on the topic or whether or not to first present the findings 'cold' and then to relate them to the literature in a separate chapter of the report. The writer favours the first approach as it seems more obvious to link the categories to previous work in the field as the categories are presented. Making the links in another chapter tends to lead to considerable repetition of information. Second, the researcher needs to consider how many verbatim examples of each category they will offer the reader. It is rarely necessary to offer every example of an item within a category and as a general rule of thumb, the presentation of three or four examples seems to be a good one. Too many examples make for tedious reading and too few examples tend to encourage the reader to question the validity of the category system.

This section has described one way of content analysing textual material using a wordprocessor. It will be noted that, although the writer used *WordPerfect*, other wordprocessors could easily be used in this context. The method described here is one way and not the only way: other approaches to content analysis are, of course, available. The aim of this approach is to encourage the researcher to use all the text that is offered to them from the respondents in a study.

You can use a shareware program to analyse textual data.

The shareware program *DT Search* is available from most shareware suppliers. Here, a method of analysing textual data using *DT Search* is described. The method is useful for any health care researcher who needs to analyse interview transcriptions or any other textual forms of data.

First, wordprocessor files containing interview transcripts are gathered together in one directory. Then, *DT Search* 'indexes' those files. That is to say, it makes a record of all the words in all the files and the order in which those words occur. Then, the researcher decides on which strings of words they wish to find in the interviews. There strings of words can be decided beforehand and this is discussed further below. Finally, *DT Search* finds every occurrence of the string of words throughout all of the interview transcripts. In this way, two important stages in data analysis have been carried out: particular phrases have been searched for and the number of times that those phrases occur has been discovered. Thus, the 'qualitative' element of the method involves deciding what sort of text to search for and what its occurrence means. This search for meaning and for subjective interpretation of the world lies at the heart of the qualitative approach to research. The 'quantitative' is the computer search for the number of occurrences of that string of text. The method is a computerized form of content analysis.

Let us imagine that a researcher has carried out unstructured interviews with ten nurses in order to explore their views about assessment and evaluation in nurse education. The interviews are all recorded onto audio tape and those recordings are transcribed on a personal computer using any wordprocessing program. Each transcript is contained within one computer file and the ten files are contained in a directory called Interview.

DT Search is asked to open a new index and the ten files in the directory called 'Interview' are marked to be included in that indexing process. *DT Search* then makes an internal list of all the words in all the transcripts and the order in which the words occur. This process takes very little time. I prepared an index of 33 interview transcripts in less than three minutes.

Next, the researcher reads through the interview transcripts and uses an adaptation of the 'open coding' process recommended in the grounded theory approach to analysing qualitative data. Using a means of highlighting the text on the screen (perhaps by using the italics function of the wordprocessor) they seek out words and phrases that are of particular interest or that seem to occur very frequently. In this way, they are preparing what has been called the 'template' approach to data analysis. The template approach involves identifying certain themes and ideas and then combing through text in a systematic way to find every occurrence of those themes and ideas. *DT Search* is particularly well placed to help in this process.

Examples of the list of words and phrases that the researcher might identify in this way are:

- summative evaluation
- student-centred learning
- student-centred approaches
- formative evaluation
- examinations
- reflection
- peer assessment
- and so on.

Clearly, the more words and phrases the researcher can generate, the richer the analysis is likely to be. On the other hand, if too many discrete phrases are identified, then the number of examples generated and counted by the program will be large and may be difficult to analyse further. Clearly, too, more complicated search strings (such as 'student-centred learning in colleges of nursing') are not likely to produce results as they represent an idiosyncratic way of using words and are unlikely to be used, in that order, by more than one person.

Finally, the *DT Search* program is instructed to 'search' for each of the strings of words. First, for example, it may be asked to search for all occurrences of the phrase 'student-centred learning' or 'peer assessment'. The program then quickly searches through each of the transcript files and produces first a listing of the number of 'hits' it has achieved, i.e. the number of times it has encountered the particular string of words. Initially, it does this with a message such as: 'Files retrieved 10; Number of hits 24'. Thus, all ten of the transcripts contain the phrase in question and the phrase occurred 24 times in total.

Next, the program can be asked to display the files containing the phrase in question and those files can be listed in any one of the following forms: unsorted; sorted by name of file; sorted by numerical name; sorted by date or sorted by 'number of hits'. The researcher may find the latter form of listing most useful. Here, the file containing the highest number of occurrences of the phrase will be listed first, then the next highest and so on. This will allow the researcher to begin to get an idea of the distribution of themes and categories throughout a series of interviews.

After this, the contents of each file may be viewed and the string of words may be viewed in context. This offers a considerable advantage over other programs which simply note the number of occurrences of a word or phrase. With *DT Search*, the context of the occurrence of a phrase can be respected and the researcher can draw out passages of text that allows them to identify what respondents felt about the particular search categories.

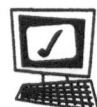

Tip

Explore statistics programs.

Qualitative research often requires the use of statistics. *C-Stat* (Cherwell) is easily installed to a hard disk. It requires *Windows 3.1.* and a 386 computer fitted with a maths coprocessor is recommended. The program is loaded to the hard disk simply by typing Install, either at the DOS prompt or via the RUN command under *Windows*.

The program opens to a spreadsheet-type screen. Data is entered as a series of rows and columns, a format familiar to anyone who has had to handle numbers. It is then a simple task to enter variable names and case names (should these be necessary). After this, the dataset is complete and can be saved to disk.

Next, particular columns or the whole dataset can be chosen for work. The program allows you to run a range of statistical routines simply by clicking on a menu. A range of descriptive statistical computations is available including the usual means, modes and frequencies. Then, a considerable list of other tests is available, including: paired-t, Wilcoxon signed rank, t-test, Mann-Whitney U and Spearman rank order. It is also possible to run multiple linear regression tests, one and two-way ANOVA, Kruskal Wallis and chi square. In essence, all the basic tests that anyone doing a small to medium quantitative study is likely to need are included here.

Results from the tests are quickly printed to the screen and these can be saved to file or printed out. The program acts quickly and runs smoothly. Context-sensitive help is available at the click of a button and this is most useful in the statistics menu. Each test is accompanied by a description and the conditions which have to be met for a particular test. It is often too easy to run statistical tests on a computer without being really clear about which ones are appropriate. This program can help you to decide which ones to choose. Obviously it could not be relied upon as the only source of decisionmaking help, but it will act as a useful memory-jogger.

Data can also be mapped out in a variety of graphical formats, including bar charts, pie charts and scattergrams. These are drawn to the screen, can be customized, saved and/or printed out. This part of the program, like all of the others, works quickly and accurately.

C-Stat for Windows is extremely easy to use. It is obvious as soon as you fire up the program what has to be done. I found it possible to create a dataset on the screen, 'analyse' that data and produce passable bar charts without recourse to the manual. When the manual is needed, it is good to note that it is clear, well written and attractive. There are plenty of worked examples and the program also comes complete with example datasets.

There are other, larger statistical programs on the market but few that can match this one for ease of use, speed and user-friendliness. It is an attractive program to work with and one that is likely to meet most researchers' needs. If you are looking for a program to organize, map and analyse your data using a range of descriptive statistics, this is the obvious choice. It is likely, too, to be useful to those whose needs are greater: its range of tests of significance is fairly broad and should satisfy most requirements. It can handle large and small datasets and most people will enjoy its 'intuitive' feel.

This will be an attractive program for many people. Health care colleges are likely to find it useful for student projects, researchers will be relieved to find a program that they can use without spending hours poring over manuals. Individual health care professionals who are working on small and larger scale research projects on undergraduate and postgraduate programs will also find it an asset. After all, there are not too many programs that you can have up and running straight out of the box.

Windows has made potentially complicated programs easy to use. *C-Stat* was (and remains) easy to use in its DOS version. In its *Windows* version it is a world-beater. It does exactly what it sets out to do and does it extremely well.

Tip

Illustrate your research reports with computer-generated graphs and charts.

Presentations (WordPerfect UK) is the *Windows* version of the already successful product *Presentations 2.0 for DOS*. That product introduced the innovation of a graphical user interface in a DOS program. This is the full *Windows* version and it is impressive. If you are a regular user of *Windows* and use a fairly powerful PC, then this may be the graphice program you need.

Initial impressions were slightly daunting. For some reason, the program takes an age to install. It comes on nine disks, which is not unusual these days. The installation process can be 'complete' – in which case the whole of the package is installed – or you can choose which elements of the program you need. Either way, installation is painfully slow. On a fast 486 computer, with plenty of memory and a fast hard disk, the process took me more than half an hour. Also, there is a general and lasting impression that the *Windows* program runs more slowly than the DOS one.

Everything else, though, is very good. *Presentations* allows you to make slides, handouts, overhead projection sheets and a range of other sorts of graphical charts and illustrations. It would be ideal for the health care professional educator who wanted a quick and easy way to produce professional-looking learning aids. It would also be of value to the researcher who needed to present data in the form of graphs, pie charts and other sorts of figures. The charting ability of the program is both easy to use and impressive.

Presentations comes with a large library containing more than 1000 editable clip art images. You have to be careful with clip art. If you use it too liberally, your work can look very home-made. Fortunately, the clip art contained with this package can be modified and edited in all sorts of ways. You can also scan in your own images and edit these in the versatile bitmap editor.

If you want to make slides (and there are numerous templates for these) you can also create a detailed set of notes to go with them. Thus, in the one package, you have the means to produce a complete conference package. A sophisticated outliner allows you to develop bullet lists and charts. Again, there is a large range of outliner templates to choose from. You can also try out various effects. If you don't like the first template you choose, you simply try another until you get the right one.

If you need help at any time, WordPerfect's Quick Tutors offer you easy tutorials at the touch of a button or the click of the mouse. This interactive way of learning the program is an excellent idea and makes learning both quick and enjoyable. Also included is a comprehensive spell checker and a thesaurus. If you use other WordPerfect programs, these facilities can be shared between them. Thus you don't have to install three or four different spell checkers but simply use the same one in a range of programs.

A copy of *Adobe Font Manager* is included with the package which gives the user a varied range of typefaces to work with. One of the important features of the *Font Manager* is its ability to load and unload fonts as they are needed. Fonts take up a lot of memory and can slow down a program. By using the *Font Manager* you only have to work with the fonts that you need.

Presentations for Windows needs a fairly powerful computer. The company suggests a minimum of a 386 processor and 4Mb of RAM. My guess is that this would be a fairly sluggish environment in which to run the program and a better configuration might be a 486 with 8Mb of RAM.

This is a professional and very practical package. The WordPerfect button bar feature means that you can customize the program to a considerable degree. Graphics and presentation programs are not ones that most people use every day. This means that there is always a risk that you will forget how to use them and have to relearn them every time you come back to the program. This seems unlikely with *Presentations*. Although most people will probably only use certain features on a regular basis, all of the functions are intuitive and it is soon obvious what you have to do once you have fired up the program after a break. This sort of ease of use, combined with highly sophisticated features, means the *PresentationsforWindows* can be useful to a wide range of health care professionals, from students to managers and from educators to researchers.

Tip

You may want to try your hand at programming.

Personal computing has changed. In the days when BBC microcom- ̨ uters held the educational sector of the market, many students who learned computing also learned to write simple programs. Indeed, the 'computing' input of a nursing course usually included a course in the BASIC language. Today, with the availability of so many commercial programs, the need for the average user to learn how to program is reduced.

On the other hand, the researcher who can program can sometimes design 'one-off' programs for a particular purpose to suit their own health care setting. They might, for example, write a database system to cope with the management of an outpatient service. A health care lecturer might write a program for storing bibliographical references, for use in educational settings. The great advantage of having pro- gramming skills is the fact that you can write exactly the program that you want. Most of us have to compromise a little with commercially written packages. This is, perhaps, most notably the case with database programs.

Whilst there is a range of programming languages to choose from, Pascal is one of the most widely used and, arguably, one of the easiest to work with.

Pascal can be used to develop a range of programs such as databases, menus, management packages and patient record systems. Pascal is high-level language which means, in essence, that the language is much easier to use than the lower level languages. Low-level languages ask you to relate very closely to the basic workings of the computer, whilst high-level languages are much more user friendly and easy to learn. In a sense, a language like Pascal resembles a crude form of human language. Each statement in a high-level language corre- sponds to several statements in a low-level language.

Developed by a European computer scientist, Nicklaus Wirth, and named after the French philosopher Blaise Pascal, early versions of Pascal were available from the early 1970s. It was designed as a teaching language and survives in this form today. The fact that 20 years have elapsed since those early versions means that the current Pascal packages are very sophisticated indeed.

Turbo Pascal for Windows (Borland) is a new version of Pascal developed especially for use under *Windows. Windows* users will be immediately at home with the sets of pull-down menus and the interface which matches that of other *Windows* programs. Also, *Turbo Pascal for Windows* can be used to develop *Windows* programs themselves. It comes with a range of detailed manuals and is, like all Borland programs, extremely well presented.

Turbo Pascal with Objects (Borland) is a much more extensive package that can allow you to do all that the *Windows* version can do and much more. 'Objects', in this case, refers to blocks of prepared code that can be incorporated into your own routines. This is version 7 of Borland's Pascal language. It is a package for any level of user, from beginners in the Pascal language to fully experienced program writers, although the sheer sophistication of the package will appeal particularly to the expert.

Some of the immediate advantages of this new version of Pascal are its ease of use – the whole package is menu driven – and its speed. This is easily the 'fastest' Pascal to date. Different colours are used to differentiate between different aspects of any program being written with this version of Pascal. This makes problem spotting easier and makes it easier for another person who might read through the text on the screen. Transfer of sections of code between different applications is also easy through a type of 'clipboard' facility that is found in *Windows*. The whole package can also be custom configured to suit the individual programmer. It is probably true to say that most average programmers will not use all of the material that is offered in this package but it is good to know that the package is comprehensive and brings the user to the cutting edge of the Pascal world. Also, as with *Turbo Pascal for Windows, Turbo Pascal with Objects* comes with a huge array of manuals, including a tutorial manual. Whilst few will be tempted to open the box and learn the whole thing from scratch on their own, this looks as though it might be possible. All of the manuals are extremely well presented and produced. One of the excellent features of this package is the amount of information that is supplied with it. You not only get the programming language: you also get a full library about that language, from a quick guide to the main features to a full set of expert user manuals.

If you are a programmer or you want to learn how to program, either of these packages will suit you well. The *Windows* version will obviously be popular with those who regularly work with *Windows*, whilst the other package represents just about the most comprehensive programming package yet produced.

RECOMMENDED READING

Foster, J.J. (1993) *Starting SPSS/PC+ and SPSS for Windows: A Beginner's Guide to Data Analysis*, 2nd edn, Sigma, Wilmslow. Available from Computer Manuals, 50 James Road, Tyseley, Birmingham B11 2BA. Telephone: 021-706-1188

Any health professional who needs to handle quantitative data soon needs a computer program to handle it. *SPSS* has been around for a long time and has been available in various versions, from mainframe to *Windows*. It is also an immensely powerful program which can handle almost any statistical test you can think of. One of the problems of such power is that it has always been a fairly complicated program to use. That was until the *Windows* version became available. Having used the DOS package for the PC and the *Windows* version, I know that I am unlikely to return to the DOS version. The *Windows* program is not only intuitive to use, it is also very attractive. You no longer need the numerous manuals that come with the program. For most of the time, at least, you can get by with the pull-down menu system. Most users are going to find that they can work out how to do descriptive statistics fairly quickly without recourse to the manual at all.

Jeremy Foster aims at doing quite a complicated task and does it very well. The two versions of SPSS are quite different to operate. The first edition of this book was all about the DOS version. For this edition, Foster has also addressed the Windows user. You can see the problem: most users will use one or the other; No one is likely to use both. This means that each type of user has to skip certain sections of the book that do not apply to them. In a sense, this makes for reduced value but in practice this turns out not to be the case. In reading the DOS sections of the book, I was reminded just how clumsy it was and made a mental note to use *Windows* versions of all programs as and when they become available – the platform is so much more approachable. Also, it was useful to remember certain functions of the DOS program and then to see how they are done in *Windows*. Thus, the 'double' approach of the book also allows you to make useful comparisons between the versions. I imagine that reading this book is likely to produce quite a few converts to *Windows*.

Foster is clearly a master of *SPSS*. He is also a talented teacher and writer. I found it possible to follow his examples both at the keyboard and by simply reading his text. This is not always the case. I have often found that computer manuals don't make a lot of sense until you have the program up and running on your computer. This makes 'bedtime reading' impossible – unless of course you take your computer to bed with you and this is unlikely to be ideal advice.

The book has a lot of chapters, 40 in all, including the appendices. This means that it is divided into short and easily digested chunks that make for accelerated reading. The early chapters introduce you to the book and to PCs and are a good guided tour. The third chapter is a simple introduction to DOS and this is followed by a straightforward introduction to *Windows*. A beginner could learn quite a lot about their computer from these initial chapters. Chapter 5 is called 'What is SPSS?' and gives a historical and descriptive overview of the program. You have to wait until Chapter 9 before you start to operate *SPSS for DOS* but by that time you feel confident enough to do so. Following chapters show you how to enter data, label it and run analyses. Chapter 15 tells you all about printing out your findings. From Chapter 17 onwards, Foster runs through the same issues but in the *Windows* version of the program. As I have suggested already, these chapters are much simpler because *SPSS for Windows* is far simpler to use.

Final chapters of the book are particularly useful. They offer a short summary of the main statistical tests and, in one, you are offered a chart to help you select the appropriate test for the sort of data you are using. One of the problems with a program like *SPSS* is that it will run almost any test on almost any data. This can lead to nonsensical results and it is vital that your data fit the criteria for the tests you are using. This is one of the clearest expositions of the way to use statistical tests that I have read. Anyone new to handling numbers is almost bound to benefit from the later chapters of this book.

The book closes with summaries of the menu structures of both sorts of programs. These are likely to be more useful to the *SPSS/PC+* user as menu structures in that program are often fairly well hidden.

One of the joys of using *Windows* is that nearly all the menu structures are the same across a range of programs.

This book is nicely produced and easy on the eye as well as being easy to read. Dr Foster is able to make his subject both interesting and accessible, talents that are not always in evidence in computer books. This is recommended to any health professional who needs to use statistics, wants to use *SPSS* and is frightened of both.

Frude, N. (1993) *A Guide to SPSS/PC+*, 2nd edn, Macmillan, London. Available from Computer Manuals, 50 James Road, Tyseley, Birmingham B11 2BA. Telephone: 021-706-1188

The Statistical Package for the Social Sciences has been around for 25 years in various forms. This book, now in its second edition, is both a guide and a tutorial to the latest DOS version. It can be used by students working alone or in organized work groups. In the later case, the lecturer can use this book as a teaching guide.

Most health professionals who do quantitative research need to crunch numbers at some point. SPSS offers them one of the most potent means of doing this and this book makes a potentially complicated program much easier to use. As in the previous edition, Neil Frude has found a way of explaining the process of entering data, analysing it and then printing out the results which should put this book on everyone's list if they are thinking about statistical analysis.

Indeed, the book is a complete introduction to handling and analysing quantitative data. The book covers the topics of collecting raw data and coding them. It then shows how to enter numerical data into the SPSS program and save the resulting files. Following chapters deal with defining the data and annotating them with descriptions and value labels. Finally, the book deals with using the dataset to produce summaries and tables and performing statistical tests.

The introduction is a particularly useful overview of the *SPSS/PC+* program itself. Also contained in the book is an example dataset. This struck me as being useful in a number of ways. First, it shows the reader how data from questionnaires and other instruments can be handled as a series of 'rows and columns'. Then it offers a set of figures to work on in the program itself. The dataset is frequently referred to throughout the text and brings the book to life.

This is more than just an introduction to a statistics program. It is also a thorough grounding in the principles of handling quantitative data. Dr Frude offers the criteria for using the various statistical tests contained in the program and this is indeed helpful. It is one thing to get a statistics package to run: it is quite another to know which tests to apply to which data.

The book closes with a glossary of statistical, computing and *SPSS/PC* terms and a guide to all of the main *SPSS/PC* commands and subcommands. Anyone coming to the program for the first time will find the book invaluable. Anyone who has used the program for some time will also find it to be a vital and necessary handbook. The program itself comes with a considerable array of manuals and none of them is as clearly written as the text of this book.

My one problem with the book is this. *SPSS/PC* is now available in a *Windows* version. That version is considerably easier to use than the previous DOS versions. Now *Windows* programs need powerful computers with lots of memory if they are to run at any speed at all (and, sometimes, if they are to run at all). Increasingly, though, it seems likely that colleges and universities making use of *SPSS/PC* will switch to the *Windows* version. This book makes no reference to the *Windows* version and is clearly addressed to a particular audience – the users of the DOS program. It is to be hoped that Dr Frude is currently working on a *Windows* version of his book. Meanwhile, this book will be of very great interest to a huge number of people still working in the DOS environment. It teaches you a great deal about handling numbers, about computers, about *SPSS* and about statistics.

Appendix
The Data Protection Act 1984.
Guideline 1: Introduction to
the Act*

1. PURPOSE OF THE ACT

Computers are in use throughout society – collecting, storing, processing and distributing information. Much of that information is about people – 'personal data' – and is subject to the Data Protection Act 1984.

The Act gives new rights to individuals about whom information is recorded on computer. They may find out information about themselves, challenge it if appropriate and claim compensation in certain circumstances. The Act places obligations on those who record and use personal data (data users). They must be open about that use (through the Data Protection Register) and follow sound and proper practices (the Data Protection Principles).

The Act is improving practice among computer users and should raise public confidence in computing. It has also allowed the United Kingdom to ratify the Council of Europe Convention on Data Protection. This should ensure that data can flow freely between the United Kingdom and other European countries which have similar laws. If the United Kingdom could not ratify the convention, other countries might wish to prevent their data being sent here. This could damage our international trade and some companies might decide to move their operations – and jobs – elsewhere.

* Reproduced with permission of the Data Protection Registrar.

2. WHAT THE ACT COVERS

The Act only applies to automatically processed information, broadly speaking, information which is processed by a computer. It does not cover information which is held and processed manually, for example, in ordinary paper files.

The Act does not cover all computerized information but only that which relates to living individuals. So, for example, it does not cover information which relates only to a company or organization and not to an individual.

Because it is dealing with a new subject, the Act uses some unfamiliar words and phrases. It is important to grasp their meaning because they define how the Act works. Guideline 2 defines them more fully but for this book the following broad description should be enough.

Personal data

Information recorded on a computer about living, identifiable individuals. Statements of fact and expressions of opinion about an individual are personal data but an indication of the data user's intentions towards the individual is not.

Data subject

An individual to whom personal data relate.

Data users

People or organizations who control the contents and use of a collection of personal data. A data user will usually be a company, corporation or other organization but it is possible for an individual to be a data user.

Computer bureaux

People or organizations who process personal data for data users or who allow data users to process personal data on their computers.

3. WHAT KINDS OF DATA ARE EXEMPT FROM THE ACT?

The Act does not apply to all personal data; data held for some purposes are exempt from the requirement to register. The Registrar cannot take enforcement action and individuals cannot exercise their rights under the Act in respect of such personal data. These exemptions are dealt with fully in Guideline 6. They cover the following situations:

- Personal data held by an individual (e.g. a home computer user in connection with personal, family or household affairs or for recreational purposes).

- Personal data used only for calculating and paying wages and pensions, keeping accounts or keeping records of purchases and sales in order to ensure that the appropriate payments are made. This exemption does not apply if the data are used for wider purposes, for example, as a personnel record or for marketing purposes.

- Personal data used for distributing articles or information to the data subjects – under this exemption only a very small amount of data can be held (usually only name and address). A data subject must be asked if they object to the data being held for this purpose. If they do object the exemption does not apply.

- Personal data held by an unincorporated members club (e.g. a sports or recreational club which is not a registered company). All the data subjects must be members of the club and must be asked if they object to the data being held for this purpose. If they object the exemption does not apply.

- Personal data which the law requires the user to make public – for example, personal data in the electoral register kept by an Electoral Registration Officer.

- Personal data which are required to be exempt to safeguard national security – whether this exemption is required is decided by a government minister.

Since these descriptions are brief, any data user who intends to rely on an exemption should read Guideline 6. Most exemptions are subject to strict conditions, particularly as to when and how information may be disclosed. In practice, many data users will find that since they cannot rely safely on the exemptions, they will need to register under the Act.

Information which is processed only for preparing the text of documents is also outside the Act's scope. This rule is sometimes referred to as the 'wordprocessor exemption'. Its effect is that the Act does not apply to information entered onto a computer with the sole purpose of editing the text and printing out a document.

4. WHAT IS IN THE REGISTER?

Every data user who holds personal data must be registered, unless all the data are exempt. Applications for registration are made on forms DPR4 and DPR1 is suitable for use by small businesses. Both forms are available from the Registrar's officer. The fee payable on an application is £75 at the date of this Guideline. The fee may change so you should check the current fee before sending in an application form.

The data user's Register entry is compiled by the Registrar from the information given in the application. The entry contains the data user's name and address together with broad descriptions of:

- the personal data which the data user holds;
- the purposes for which the data are used;
- the sources from which the data user intends to obtain the information;
- the people to whom the data user may wish to disclose the information;
- any overseas countries or territories to which the data user may wish to transfer the personal data.

The Registrar can refuse registration applications, for example, if they contain insufficient information.

Computer bureaux which process personal data for others must also register. Their Register entries will contain only their name and address.

Data users and computer bureaux may apply at any time to alter or cancel their Register entries.

Data users and computer bureaux who should register but have not commit a criminal offence.

Registered data users commit a criminal offence if they knowingly or recklessly operate outside the descriptions contained in their Register entries. So, for example, it would be an offence to hold personal data of a type not described in the Register entry.

The Register is open to public inspection at the Registrar's office in Wilmslow. Inspection of the Register is free. Official copies of individual Register entries (known as 'certified copies') are available from the Registrar's office. A fee of £2 per entry is payable.

5. THE DATA PROTECTION PRINCIPLES

Registered data users must comply with the Data Protection Principles in relation to the personal data they hold. The Principles are dealt with in detail in Guideline 4. Broadly they state that personal data shall:

- be obtained and processed fairly and lawfully;
- be held only for the lawful purposes described in the Register entry;
- be used only for those purposes and only be disclosed to those people described in the Register entry;
- be adequate, relevant and not excessive in relation to the purpose for which they are held;
- be accurate and, where necessary, kept up to date;
- be held no longer than is necessary for the registered purpose;
- be surrounded by proper security.

The Principles also provide for individuals to have access to data held about themselves and, where appropriate, to have the data corrected or deleted.

To enforce compliance with the Principles, the Registrar can serve three types of notice. They are:

1. an enforcement notice, requiring the data user to take specified action to comply with the particular Principle. Failure to comply with the notice would be a criminal offence;

2. a deregistration notice, cancelling the whole or part of a data user's Register entry. The data user would then be committing an offence if it continued to treat the personal data subject to the notice as though they were registered;

3. a transfer prohibition notice, preventing the data user from transferring personal data overseas if the Registrar is satisfied that the transfer is likely to lead to a Principle being broken. Failure to comply with such a notice is a criminal offence.

A person on whom a notice is served is entitled to appeal against the Registrar's decision to the Data Protection Tribunal.

6. WHAT RIGHTS DO INDIVIDUALS HAVE?

The Act give new legal rights to individuals (data subjects) concerning personal data held about them.

Compensation

A data subject is entitled to seek compensation through the courts if, after 11 September 1984, damage has been caused by the loss, unauthorized destruction or unauthorized disclosure of the personal data. If damage is proved, then the Court may also order compensation for any associated distress.

'Unauthorized' means without the authority of the data user or computer bureau concerned.

A data subject may also seek compensation through the courts for damage caused after 10 May 1986 by inaccurate data. Again compensation for distress may be awarded if damage can be proved.

Correction or deletion

If personal data are inaccurate the data subject may complain to the Registrar or apply to the courts for correction or deletion of the data.

Subject access

An individual is entitled, on making a written request, to be supplied by any data user with a copy of any personal data held about him or her. The data user may charge a fee of up to £10 for supplying this information from one Register entry.

This right is called the 'subject access right'. Sometimes the right will not apply – for example, where giving subject access would be likely to prejudice the prevention or detection of crime. Those occasions are set out in Guideline 6 under the heading 'Subject Access Exemptions'. Usually a request for subject access must be responded to within 40 days. If it is not, the data subject is entitled to complain to the Registrar or to apply to the courts for an order that the data user should give access.

Complaint to the Registrar

A data subject who considers there has been a breach of one of the Principles or any other provision of the Act is entitled to complain to the Data Protection Registrar. If the complaint raises a matter of substance, is made without undue delay and directly affects the complainant, the Registrar must consider it. If the complaint is justified and cannot be resolved informally then the Registrar may use his powers to prosecute or to serve one of the notices already mentioned. In any event, when the Registrar has considered the complaint, he must notify the complainant of any action which he proposes to take.

7. WHEN MAY PERSONAL DATA BE DISCLOSED?

The Act does not prevent a data user from disclosing information about an individual if the user wishes to do so. Disclosures may be made if either:

- the person to whom the disclosure is made is described in the disclosures section of the data user's Register entry; or
- the disclosure is covered by one of the 'non-disclosure exemptions'. They are described in detail in Guideline 6 and include, for example, disclosures required by law or made with the data subject's consent.

There is therefore no general right for the data subject to object to the disclosure of personal data relating to him or her. However, the first Data Protection Principle does require data users to obtain information fairly and they should be careful not to deceive or mislead anyone about the purpose for which the information is to be held, used or disclosed.

The compensation rules mentioned in section 6 apply only to 'unauthorized' disclosures, meaning those made without the authority of the data user or computer bureau concerned. Unless a non-disclosure exemption applies computer bureaux may only disclose personal data with the authority of the data user who controls the data.

8. WHAT DOES THE DATA PROTECTION REGISTRAR DO?

The Data Protection Registrar is an independent officer who is appointed by the Queen and who reports directly to Parliament. His duties are to:

- establish the Register of data users and computer bureaux and make it publicly available;
- spread information on the Act and how it works;
- promote compliance with the Data Protection Principles;
- encourage, where appropriate, the development of codes of practice to help data users to comply with the Principles;
- consider complaints about breaches of the Principles or the Act and, where appropriate, prosecute offenders or service notices on registered data users and computer bureaux who are breaking the Principles.

9. THE DATA PROTECTION TRIBUNAL

The Data Protection Tribunal consists of a legally qualified chairman together with lay members. The lay members are appointed to represent the interests of data users and data subjects. The Tribunal's task is to consider appeals by data users or computer bureaux against the Registrar's decisions. Appeals may relate to the refusal of a registration application or to the service of an enforcement, deregistration or transfer prohibition notice. The Tribunal can overturn the Registrar's decision and substitute whatever decision it thinks fit. On questions of law there is a further appeal from the Tribunal to the High Court.

References

Acerson, K.L. (1992) *Guide To WordPerfectforWindows*, Ziff-Davis, Emeryville, California.

Arnold, J.M. and Pearson, G.A. (eds) (1992) *Computer Applications in Nursing Education and Practice*, National League for Nursing, New York.

Edelhart, M. (1992) *PC Computing's '2001 Windows Tips'*, Ziff-Davis, Emeryville, California.

Gann, R. (1993) The ultimate Windows upgrade? *What Personal Computer*, December.

Gookin, D. (1993) *Microsoft Guide to Optimizing Windows*, Microsoft Press, Redmond, Washington.

Kennedy, R.C. (1993) Pentiums are fast – but no panacea. *Windows Magazine*, November.

Kilby, S.A. and McAlindon, M.N. (1992) Searching the literature yourself: why, how and what to search, in *Computer Applications in Nursing Education and Practice*, (eds J.M. Arnold and G.A. Pearson), National League for Nursing, New York.

Magee, M. (1993) Counter attack. *Computer Buyer*, October.

Moss, J. (1993) The direct guide to portable PCs. *PC Direct*, April.

Nicholson, M. (1993) Inside Windows. *PC Plus*, November.

Norfolk, D. (1993) Protect and survive. *PC Plus*, December.

Norfolk, D. (1994) Lock up your data. *PC Plus*, January.

Robertson, D. (1993) Configuration station. *Windows Magazine*, November.

Stephens, M. (1993) The happy shopper. *Windows User*, December.

Stephens, M. (1994) *TNT or OTT? Windows User*, January.

Stobie, I. (1994) *Speedier media. What PC?* January.

Venditto, G. (1992) *PC Magazine Guide to Using Windows 3.1*, Ziff-Davis, Emeryville, California.

Waddilove, R. (1992) Making the move. *PC Today*, July.

Windows User (1993) Back to basics. August.

Index